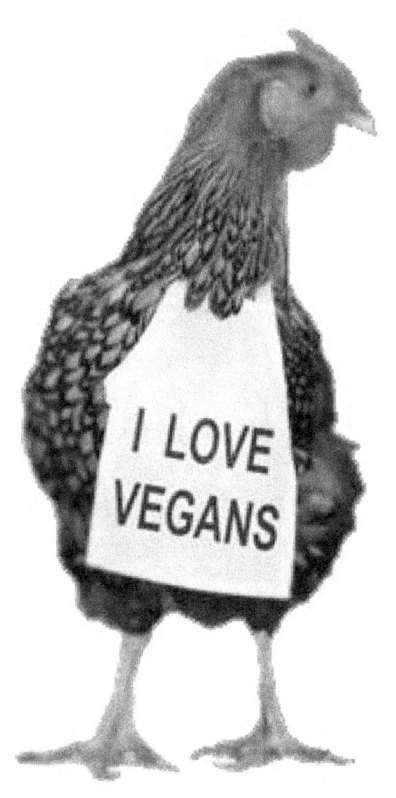

The Essential Vegan

The No-Nonsense Guide to a Vegan Lifestyle
for Better Health and Happiness

Christina Summers

Contents

Introduction

When I became vegan in April 2011, I had no clue what I was doing. Despite cooking healthy before becoming vegan, for some reason it felt like starting all over again. Let me tell you, though, it was the best decision I made for my health and happiness. The goal of this book is to provide you with the down and dirty information to transition into becoming vegan YOUR way. I realize everyone is unique and has different strengths and challenges with food. I am providing you with an arsenal of practical information about veganism and how to overcome common obstacles you may face in the world, from friends and family and in your own kitchen.

Becoming vegan is tough enough so I wrote this book in a way that is easy to follow and understand. By the time you finish this book there are a few things I want you to walk away with. I want you to be confident knowing that you CAN do this at whatever pace you choose, which ever phase of the transition is just where you need to be. I aim for you to learn a few things about health and how being vegan affects not only your personal health but also the health of the environment and billions of animals in the world.

Before we dive into the book you may be wondering what exactly is vegan? According to the dictionary.com, a vegan is "a person who refrains from using any animal product whatever for food, clothing or any purpose." To me, being vegan is living a life in a conscious manner that causes the least amount of pain, suffering or discomfort to all beings in the world. I choose to not consume any meat or animal products, wear animal clothing, or use personal products that were tested on animals. What does being or becoming vegan mean to you?

There are a variety of reasons to become vegan. You will

impact countless human and animal lives just by choosing what you put on your plate. It is a powerfully beautiful feeling knowing that because you chose to not eat meat you have saved animal lives, lessened CO_2 emissions and contribution to deforestation of the rainforest, and your body is not being clogged with animal fat. I chose to become vegan for ethical reasons. Sometimes it may seem easier, especially when traveling, to pick up something not vegan for the sake of convenience; however, this book will teach you what to do in these situations so you can stay on your vegan path.

Another great reason to become vegan, which I experienced, was an increase in my overall health. It was difficult for me to find my balance at first, which I will go into detail later in the book. Once I found my happy balance I feel like an unstoppable force. I have energy all day long, which is something I had never experienced before. I am able to exercise for a longer amount of time, and I am stronger than ever. Also I am healthy as an ox at my doctor checkups.

The final reason I am vegan is for the environment. There are so many different aspects of the environment, from the drinking water to the air quality, which you help improve by choosing to become vegan. I want you to think for a moment, what is your reason for wanting to become vegan? Do you want to help not only farm animals but animals all over the world? Do you want to lower your cholesterol and get off your medications? Do you want to improve the environment by cutting out meat in your diet? If you answered yes to any of these, keep on reading to learn how easy it can be to thrive, be strong and be happy on a vegan lifestyle.

Vegan Basics

The Vegan Kitchen

This has to be the most overwhelming part of transitioning to a vegan diet, converting the kitchen. I transformed my kitchen gradually. When I was running out of groceries and needed to make a trip to the store I replaced my typical dairy products with their coconut, almond or soy counterparts. Instead of purchasing milk I bought almond milk. By gradual changes I found the transition to be less daunting and easier on the wallet. Now I will warn you, on your first trip to the store since becoming vegan you will spend a lot of time looking at all of the new products you have to choose from. That's OK, it's fun...but I don't recommend taking young children with you on that particular trip. The next week I went through my pantry and replace any refined grains such as white pasta or white rice with brown rice or whole grain pasta.

The following sections are items I recommend having in your kitchen on a regular basis.

Pantry

I like to have on hand a variety of dry and canned beans such as garbanzo, black, adzuki and pinto beans. It is also important to have an array of nuts and seeds including walnuts, pecans, pepitas, hemp seeds, chia seeds and flax meal. When ridding your pantry of refined grains, such as white rice, white breads, white flours, you can replenish it with a wide variety of whole grains such as brown rice, millet, amaranth, quinoa and farro. Dry fruit is important to have on hand because you can sweeten baked goods and smoothies naturally; my favorites are dried cherries, cranberries, coconut flakes and dates. Some other grains to have in stock are breakfast grains such as rolled oats and steel cut oats. When cooking I find that spices make all the difference in the final product. Spices have the ability to turn a dish from good to *bam, that's good*! Last but not least, especially for bakers out there, different types of flours are good to have around including whole wheat flour, whole wheat pastry flour and spelt flour.

Fridge

I absolutely love the look and feel of a refrigerator fully stocked with beautiful colors of different fruits and vegetables. It is crucial as a new vegan to widen your horizons of fruits and vegetables to eat. To this day I continue to learn and discover new fruits and veggies. Can you believe I never had a butternut squash until a few years ago?! So stock your fridge with the colors of the rainbow!

Going back to seasoning your food with spice, condiments also play a big role in making vegan food awesome. My favorites are hummus, Vegenaise and whole grain mustard. So I will admit that I am obsessed with nut butters, especially almond butter, peanut butter and cashew butter. The reason nut butters are listed under fridge is because nuts spoil much quicker in the pantry than in the fridge. Rather than non-dairy milk, you will typically find almond milk and coconut milk in my fridge. I also love to have a protein source like tempeh or tofu in my fridge.

Freezer

My freezer is quite lame, to be honest. I recommend having frozen fruits to throw into smoothies or even for a snack. Frozen veggies are also great to have around that you can throw into some boiling water for a couple minutes and voila! Something you will always find in my freezer is frozen bananas to throw in my smoothies or make banana soft-serve. For fuss-free meals I like to keep some organic frozen veggie patties to top salads with, or to throw in wraps or burger buns. What freezer isn't complete without coconut ice cream for a little indulgence? My favorite brand of coconut ice cream is Luna and Larry's Coconut Bliss.

Must Have Equipment

There are certain tools that I don't know how I lived my life without. A high-power blender such as a Vitamix is critical to have in your kitchen; it will transform your life. You can whip up salsa effortlessly, smoothies in seconds and silky smooth soups so fast. My favorite tool, even more than the Vitamix, is an immersion blender. Basically an immersion blender is a hand-held blender that you can stick into soup pots and make creamy soups without having to transfer to a blender. A food processor is also a very handy small appliance to have around to make nut butters, homemade flours, banana soft-serve and so much more. Two little hand-held tools I dig are the microplane and potato masher. I use the microplane to zest citrus, and grate ginger and garlic very finely. The potato masher just makes mashing potatoes super easy, and I like super easy.

Dictionary

Soy Products

Tempeh: Tempeh is the king of the soy products in my book! You can find tempeh in most grocery stores nowadays by the refrigerated tofu. Warning: When you first see this in the package you may think it kind of looks like brains in block form. Don't freak out! The reason it looks this way is because it is the actual soybean in a fermented state. Aside from the actual soybean, tempeh is the most whole form of soy. The fermentation binds the soybeans together to make that funky block.

Since tempeh is a fermented soy product it is an excellent source of probiotics, helping keep your gut happy. Tempeh is also a wonderful source of protein. When purchasing tempeh, make sure to check the date on the package, and look for tempeh that has no dark spotting on it. Like its brother, tofu, tempeh takes on the flavors of whatever you season it with. My favorite way to prepare tempeh is to slice into strips and let it marinate in your favorite sauce overnight in the fridge.

TVP (Textured Vegetable Protein): Sounds freaky, right? I would rather it was called powdered soy or dried soy. Anyways, TVP really is just soybeans that have been cooked under pressure and then dried. The dry texture is kind of like coarse ground flour. Once added to liquid it plumps up within a few minutes, making it a super duper addition to soups to give some oomph.

TVP provides an excellent source of pure plant protein, so if you are concerned about getting enough protein in your diet this is an easy way to do it. You can find TVP in the bulk section of many groceries; also the Bob's Red Mill brand sells it.

Tofu: Glorious tofu! Before all of these cool products came out on the market for vegans there was tofu. Tofu has gotten a bad rap lately, such as an increased risk of breast cancer.. Studies on laboratory animals taking soy *supplements* have mixed results on breast cancer. Human studies show no link between consuming soy and breast cancer. I personally think if you purchase quality Certified Organic, Non-GMO tofu you will be just fine. However, I also condone doing your own research to decide if incorporating tofu in your diet is a good choice. Tofu has been a go-to for vegans forever because it is high in protein and calcium. Tofu is a chameleon; it takes on whatever flavors you put on it. You can prepare tofu in all the ways you prepare meat; BBQ, grill, sauté, bake, and fry. Although I am not a fan of fried foods, it is an option.

Tamari: Very similar to soy sauce, tamari is a rich-tasting soy sauce. The main difference between the two is that tamari is made with very little to no wheat and an increased amount of soybeans lending its rich flavor. This goes great in any kind of Asian-inspired sauce like my peanut dipping sauce.

Miso paste: Miso is basically a fancy Japanese term for fermented soy paste. The longer the paste ferments, the darker in color and deeper in taste it becomes. I use miso paste in place of salt in numerous dishes.

Whole Grains

A complex carbohydrate is a term thrown around a lot lately, but not everyone knows what that really means. A complex carb is one where three or more sugars are linked together in a chain. These sugars are filled with vitamins, minerals and fiber. Due to their complexity they take longer to digest, keeping us fuller longer and stabilizing our blood sugar level. All of the grains in this book are complex carbohydrates.

Steel cut oats: These little guys pack a big nutritional punch! They are the most whole form of the oh-so-popular quick instant oats. They are chewier and nuttier and oh so delicious! Because they are a whole grain and full of fiber they are slowly digested, keeping your blood sugar stable and helping you feel full for hours. Bring ¼ cup oats and 1 cup water to a boil; let them dance together for about 20 minutes. Top with some nuts and fruits and you are set!

Rolled oats: These bad boys are definitely my go-to in the winter here in Colorado. They provide the same nutrients as its steel cut brother but take half the cooking time.

Farro: The first time I had farro was at a pizza joint in Fort Worth, TX, after kicking ass at the Mud Run! Eating this was a turning point in my grain adventures. Farro is an "ancient grain" coming to the states from Italy and is chock full of B vitamins, especially B3, and minerals such as zinc and manganese. This grain will give you sustained energy and a full feeling for hours.

Quinoa: Man, this little guy sure has been getting a lot of attention lately, and for good reason! Did you know that quinoa is not a grain but actually a seed? This little one is so easy to prepare in about 20 minutes you can enjoy some fluffy goodness packed with all of the essential amino acids making this a complete protein. This is a staple in my pantry year round; quinoa is great as a breakfast grain, stirred in soups, in burritos, on top of salads, anywhere really!

Amaranth: This little grain is also one of those ancient grains that the Aztecs used as a staple in their diet. Amaranth has some unique characteristics by containing lysine and amino acids not typically found in grains. You can simmer the grain and enjoy like porridge; you can also toast it in a dry skillet to enjoy a nice crunchy nutty flavor. This grain is a bit more difficult to find in the grocery but check the bulk section or Bob's Red Mill packages.

Millet: Millet is less difficult to find than amaranth and is super versatile! You can either make the texture crunchy by toasting it, or creamy by boiling it. My favorite way to enjoy millet is by toasting 1 cup for about 3 minutes in a teaspoon of coconut oil, then adding add 2 ½ cups water, broth or milk and bringing to a boil. Reduce the heat, cover and simmer for about 20 minutes until the water is absorbed.

Sprouted grains: Sprouted grains increase the grains' nutrients such as vitamin B, vitamin C, folate and fiber. Sprouted grains are also less allergenic to those with grain sensitivities. My favorite sprouted bread brand is Ezekiel.

Condiments

Nutritional yeast: It was love at first bite. Your mellow yellow color, cheesy smell and taste. From the first time I sprinkled you on a salad and then made vegan cheese with you as the star. Nutritional yeast, you rock my vegan B12 world! You may hear nutritional yeast referred to as "nooch." I'm not sure why they call it that but it took me nearly a year to realize that they were the same thing. When shopping for this be sure to buy nutritional yeast, NOT brewer's yeast, which will taste like crap. Another reason besides its rockin' cheese flavor is that it is also fortified with vitamin B12, which is essential for the body and is primarily found in animal meats.

Hummus: Oh, hummus how I love thee. Almost every vegan will have either store-bought or homemade hummus in their fridge at all times. Hummus is simply chickpeas (garbanzo beans), lemon, tahini and seasonings. My favorite way to eat hummus is as a dip for veggies and even apples! I also will slather it on sandwiches.

Apple cider vinegar: OK, guys, I have used a couple different brands and by far Braggs Apple Cider Vinegar is the best out there. ACV has what's called the "mother"; the mother is an enzyme strand of protein molecules with living nutrients and bacteria. Be sure to dilute the ACV in some water because it is very acidic and can damage your teeth if drank straight. Some highlights of ACV is that it is high in potassium, helps your body maintain a healthy pH level due to its alkaline properties, regulates blood pressure and aids in digestion.

I make myself a little ACV drink every morning simply combining 12-16 oz warm water, 1 Tbs ACV, ½ lemon and a smidge of agave nectar. My bowels swear by this drink. I also had tremendous luck with ACV clearing up any skin problems by putting a dab directly on the problem area overnight.

Coconut oil: This is my oil obsession! I used to be so scared of fat growing up, bombarded with all of those fat-free claims. Man...healthy fats rock my world now! This is a unique oil because it is a medium chain triglyceride (MCT) providing your body with energy! I love stirring coconut oil in some hot steamy oats, tossed in smoothies and used in veggie sautés.

Blackstrap molasses: A healthful sweetener that has numerous minerals including iron which many times is lacking in a vegan diet. In order to reap the full benefits of the iron it is best taken with vitamin C for absorption. This is a very thick syrup adding a robust bittersweet flavor to gingerbread.

Whole grain mustard: Did you know that mustard seed contains phytonutrients, which help to battle cancer cells? It is also helpful to those with arthritis due to its high amount of selenium and magnesium. I love whole-grain mustard paired with creamy avocado.

Vegan Protein

Legumes: Legumes for years were a mystery to me. Is it a bean? Is it lentils? What the heck is a legume?! By definition a legume is a pod such as a bean that splits in two valves with the seeds attached to one edge of the valve. Under the legume umbrella are beans, peas, lentils and peanuts. They are rich in calcium, protein, fiber and folate.

Beans

Beans were a veggie I had to learn to like; now I can't get enough of them. There are tons of different varieties of beans. Not only are beans full of protein and antioxidants, they are also full of fiber. One cup of beans provides half your recommended amount of fiber for the day. As you can tell it is very easy to get enough fiber on a well-balanced vegan diet. One of my favorite ways to enjoy beans is to bake a sweet potato and load that sucka up with beans, spices, nutritional yeast, salsa and avocado.

Which is better for you canned or dry beans? From a nutritional standpoint dry and canned beans are the same. However canned beans can have added salt so you want to be sure to rinse and drain your beans before eating. Dry beans require for them to be soaked in water overnight and boiled for at least 10 minutes. Boiling is crucial in preparing dry beans because beans by nature can be toxic and cause food poisoning if not prepared properly. My vote, I most always go with organic canned beans that are in cans that have BPA free lining.

Fun side note: the larger the beans the larger the toots...if you are trying to impress a hot date stick to the smaller beans like black and adzuki.

Top Bean Picks

Black beans

Garbanzo/Chickpeas

Pinto beans

Adzuki beans

Cannellini beans

Kidney beans

Lentils

Remember the legume family? Well, the lentil is a member of that fine family. So I had never tried a lentil before becoming vegan and man, was I ever missing out! Chock full of cholesterol-lowering fiber and blood-boosting iron!

Types of Lentils

Brown Lentils: The most common found in stores, these lentils hold their shape pretty well when cooked and can be added to a variety of different dishes.

French Green or Puy Lentils: Also quite common and originally grown in Le Puy, France, these fancy little green lentils take a bit longer to cook but keep their shape well; they also have a bit more of a crunch to them than the brown ones.

Red Lentils: These delicate lentils turn golden in color when cooked and also get mushy when cooked, so they go great in purees. You can even disguise them in baked goods for a protein punch!

Cooking Lentils

The best way I found to cook lentils is to first rinse the lentils picking out any pebbles that may have joined then combine 1 cup lentils, 2 cups water and bring to a boil; once boiling lower heat to a small simmer and cook uncovered for 20-30 minutes. If lentils still feel crunchy add some more water to just cover the lentils. Keep them in your fridge all week and toss on salads, in soups or even in wraps and pasta dishes.

Vegan Protein Powder

There is a HUGE selection of vegan protein powders on the market right now. There are a variety of vegan protein sources from hemp protein, brown rice protein, soy protein and blends of all of them. I have tried quite a few and straight up the best ones in my opinion are SunWarrior and Vega. These two brands mix well with water or milk and go fabulous in smoothies. I use these very sparingly because they are not whole foods, which is how I prefer to get my protein. I use these when I know I won't have the opportunity to get good quality protein in my system that day.

Nuts & Seeds

Tahini: Tahini is basically just ground sesame seeds. It has been used in Mediterranean cooking for ages. Tahini is a main ingredient in making hummus!

Almond butter: My. Vegan. Food. Obsession. Growing up, my favorite food was ice cream; well, watch out ice cream there is a new creamy scrumptious food in town...ALMOND BUTTER! Filled with essential vitamins and minerals like vitamin E, protein and fiber, 1-2 Tbs a day keeps my active body and curious taste buds happy.

Cashew butter: If I am in the mood for healthy creamy yet milder flavor nut butter I reach for cashew butter. Cashews are masters of disguise and go excellent in homemade cheese, and even go great when making a sweet cashew cream for dessert.

Peanut butter: Most everyone knows of peanut butter, did you know that eanut butter is the highest in protein of all its fellow nut butter buddies? There are a couple of misconceptions about this protein powerhouse. 1. Peanuts are not nuts, they are actually in the legume family. 2. Many people think there is actual dairy butter in it, there is not. 3.

Chia seeds: BAM! Chia seeds are rock stars to endurance athletes and vegans. Know those little chia pets in commercials from the 90s? Chia seeds are how those little dudes grow. Before the chia pet craze these seeds were used by the people living in the Andes Mountains. They used them to stay full and stay energized all day. Chia seeds are full of Omega-3 fatty acids (learn the importance of Omega-3 fatty acids in Chapter 4: How to Be a Healthy Vegan), protein and fiber. They plump up in liquid, which can come in handy when making an egg replacement or a pudding.

Flax seeds: Flax seeds are high in Omega-3 Fatty Acids which are crucial for a healthy body. Be sure when you consume flax seed that they are ground. If you eat flax seeds whole they will just pass on through you and not be absorbed. You can either buy pre-ground flax seed or use a coffee grinder if you have whole flax.

Hemp seeds: Yeah, man...hemp seeds. Despite their name these hemp seeds come from the male cannabis plant, which is the one that does NOT make you high because it does not contain THC which is the chemical that gets people high. The male plant is used for clothing fibers and hemp seeds. Hemp seeds are a complete protein like quinoa, just meaning that they contain all of the essential amino acids. I like to toss hemp seeds on top of cereal, in smoothies, in baked goods even to make quick milk!

Miscellaneous

Dates: These delicious tropical fruits are found in American grocery stores dried. They are an excellent source of vitamin A, iron and dietary fiber. I love to use dates as a natural sweetener in smoothies, nut milks and in raw desserts.

Coconut cream: This is simply the cream that rises to the top of the coconut milk. Coconuts including the cream are vital in stabilizing blood sugar and lowering cholesterol. You can even make your own healthy whipped cream.

Sauerkraut: Most of us are familiar with this sour condiment on Reuben sandwiches. Sauerkraut is fermented cabbage. Sauerkraut as well as all other fermented veggies is full of probiotics, which are crucial to a healthy gut. I used to despise this stuff; I finally found one that I dig, Bubbies. If you've never tried it before, try putting some in a dry skillet and warming through a bit. I find this brings out a lovely flavor and is not so intense on the sourness.

Non-dairy cheese: Now, I know this book is about becoming vegan without the reliance of faux products. I do, however, also understand that dairy is one of the toughest things for people to give up. When you have a cheese craving, Daiya is a killer replacement. It is stretchy, melty and tasty. Made from flour and oils, this vegan cheese comes in shreds in a variety of flavors, slices for sandwiches, and cheese wedges.

Sprouts

There are many different types of sprouts; alfalfa, broccoli, clover, radish and more. These little guys are packed full of essential nutrients such as vitamins A, C, B1, B6. They are also easier to digest, helping reduce bloating which can happen when transitioning to a vegan diet. I like to throw sprouts in smoothies and juices, and on top of salads and soups.

Bean sprouts: High in vitamin A, mung bean sprouts have long white shoots with small yellow leaves. These go great in stir-frys, soups and salads.

Green leafy sprouts: These are my favorite sprouts; they are long and thin with dark green leaves at the ends.

Alfalfa sprouts: Most common in stores, alfalfa sprouts go excellent in wraps and sandwiches.

Radish sprouts: Small and spicy, they go great in salads.

Sunflower sprouts*:* Similar to alfalfa sprouts, these have a mild sweet flavor.

Quick Recipes

Tempeh Bacon

Ingredients:

1 block tempeh cut into strips

1 Tbs tamari or soy sauce

1 Tbs grade b maple syrup

1 tsp EVOO

Couple splashes liquid smoke

Splash of ACV (apple cider vinegar)

Garlic powder, chili powder, paprika, salt and pepper

Directions:

Let marinate 2 hours or overnight. Heat a skillet over medium heat with olive oil. Heat the tempeh 3-4 minutes each side and get ready to have your mind blown!

Vegan Soft-Serve

Ingredients:

2 frozen bananas chopped

Couple splashes of almond milk

Directions:

In a food processor, blend up the nanners and milk until creamy. Feel free to add any yummies like fruit, nut butters, jams, etc.

Vegan Kitchen Transformation Startup Kit

Take this quiz to find out if you need the Beginner, Medium or Advanced starter kit! Now, be honest with this quiz. This is for you so start by being honest with yourself and I can help.

1. How many packaged foods do you have in your kitchen including the pantry, fridge and freezer?
   a. 0-5
   b. 6-9
   c. 10-1,000,000,000

2. Look at the packaged foods; do they contain animal products (casein, whey, eggs, whole, part or skim milk powder)?
   a. No
   b. About half
   c. Majority

3. Look in your fridge; how many animal meat or by-products do you have – remember this includes all dairy (cheese, milk, yogurt, butter)?
   a. 0-2 items
   b. 3-5 items
   c. Holy crap this thing is full of meat, dairy & eggs

4. Do you feel overwhelmed with how much you need to replace?
   a. Nah, I got this
   b. I can get rid of most but I really love my ice cream
   c. I want to cry

Point Values A = 2 B = 4 C = 6

Time for the results...drum rolllllll!

1-10 I Piss Greens

10-20 Carrot Head

20-30 New Vegger

During my transition to full vegan I was vegetarian for three months. Although I ate healthy before, I felt like my world turned upside down. I never realized how vegetables, grains, legumes and fruits can truly be the show-stoppers of a meal. It may seem like a bit of information overload to learn new terms and buy ingredients you are not used to. Approach this with a playful, creative, fun and forgiving way and you will not have a problem. I say forgiving because there is so much to learn you may slip up now and then when eating something only to realize after you ate it that it contained milk or eggs.

We all make mistakes, but don't get discouraged, all you can do is power on and learn from your mistake. You may realize during this vegan kitchen clean-up that a lot of what you already have is vegan—awesome, that will make things easier. Others may notice that a lot of what is in the kitchen is not vegan, and that's cool too, because you have so much new stuff to discover and taste!

NEW VEGGER

Pantry

Remove all of the packaged foods you have in the pantry that contain animal products. Some common milk derivatives found in packaged foods are casein, whey, caseinates, any form of milk powders. Remove these first. Afterwards check out the remaining packaged foods on the shelf. Now, pick 2 that you LOVE and get rid of the rest. The goal here is not to throw away all of your foods but to replace them with wonderful homemade versions.

I realize that this may take some time to do or may not be financially feasible. If this is the case finish the packages you have and next time you go to replace them, replace with a vegan version.

Buy the following for your now naked pantry: 4 different types of beans, brown rice, cashews, walnuts, 1 nut butter of choice, quinoa, nutritional yeast, spices other than salt and pepper.

Fridge

There really is not a whole lot of give or take here. If you have meat, dairy or eggs these need to be removed. Luckily these days there are plenty of wonderful dairy alternatives. Refer to the swap chart for my top picks of dairy replacements! I highly recommend purchasing some tempeh and tofu; you can also buy shelf-stable tofu but I prefer organic water-packed.

DAIRY & EGG SWAP CHART

Cheese	Daiya cheese shreds, slices, wedges
Dairy milk	Almond, soy, rice, hemp or coconut milk
Butter	Earth Balance butter spread, coconut oil, extra virgin olive oil
Yogurt	So Delicious coconut yogurt
Coffee Creamer	So Delicious coffee creamer
Eggs	Tofu scramble
Ice cream	Luna and Larry's Coconut Bliss Ice Cream
Mayonnaise	Vegenaise
Cream cheese	Tofutti cream cheese

GRAIN SWAP CHART

White rice	Brown rice, quinoa
Quick cooking oats	Whole rolled oats, steel cut oats
White flour	Whole wheat flour (oat, pastry),all-purpose unbleached flour, spelt flour,

SUGAR SWAP CHART

White sugar	Organic sugar, maple syrup, coconut sugar, agave, brown rice syrup

MEAT SWAP CHART

Hamburgers	Portobello mushrooms, veggie patties, preferably homemade but Amy's veggies patties are good
Sausage	Field Roast Sausages (Italian, Apple Sage, Chorizo)
Bacon	Tempeh Bacon

CARROT HEAD

Pantry

Yo, so maybe you already have the packaged foods out of your pantry and have a few beans up in there. Let's add some more vegan goodness to that pantry!

Try even more new beans! I found these butter beans (no, there's no butter in them) and they were super good!

Try out the red or green lentils.

Variety of nuts—variety is the spice of life, right? Try some uncommon but oh-so-tasty nuts like Brazil nuts, pine nuts, or macadamia nuts.

Variety of seeds—seeds tend to get overlooked, at least at my house. Buy some sunflower seeds, ground flax seed or sesame seeds.

Antioxidant-boosting spices such as turmeric, cinnamon, cayenne pepper.

Fridge

Let's take a look at that fridge. No meat, check! No dairy, check! No eggs, check! Let's broaden the variety of fruits and veggies up in there. Each trip you make to the grocery pick up something you normally would not touch. Like celery root, have you seen how fugly one of those are?! Well, pick one up because they are amazingly scrumptious. Their delicate flavor and silky smooth texture is perfect in place of mashed taters.

I PISS GREENS

Pantry

You are a veggie-loving freakazoid! So awesome for you! No bags of food up in your pantry. No meat in your kitchen. Dairy, please, that is long gone. Eggs, don't even miss them. Well, where to go from here? Superfood that kitchen up!

- Add superfoods like goji berries to your pantry; my favorite brand is Dragon Herbs Goji Berries

- Get your chlorophyll on and pick up some spirulina or chlorella algae to mix into your smoothies for a super green boost of energy and increase oxygen to your blood.

- Chia seeds may be pricey but are well worth the money.

Fridge

In the fridge let's get creative with fresh herbs such as cilantro, sage, flat-leaf parsley, rosemary and so many more! It is amazing how herbs can completely transform a dish.

In the freezer throw in some acai berry smoothie packs. The acai berry is from the Amazon and is filled with antioxidants and omega-3 fatty acids.

Become Vegan Your Way

When becoming vegan you basically have two options; cold turkey or transitional vegan. There are advantages and challenges to both methods. This chapter will cover how to transition both ways and how to overcome challenges of both methods, and provide tips for a successful transition for new vegans. Here we go!

Cold Turkey

There are some people who totally rock at making life-changing decisions by going cold turkey. I give mad props to you guys! If cold turkey is typically your style that is bad ass! There are some definite advantages and challenges that come with this transition.

Advantages

You make up your mind and stick to your plan, and you are immediately making an impact on your health.

You will most likely lose quite a bit of weight faster than if you keep some animal products in your diet.

You will get to eat a lot of whole plant foods.

You will experience increased energy.

Challenges

Restock an entire kitchen with vegan alternatives.

OVERCOME! Before going cold turkey, go through the swap list provided in the book and have these items ready to swap. Consider donating non-vegan food to a food bank, or a neighbor.

You feel you are not getting enough nutrients

OVERCOME! Do your research beforehand and talk with other vegans and vegetarians for advice before making the switch. You need to do sufficient nutrition research, which you will learn about in later chapters. Before becoming vegan to make sure you are prepared with foods to ensure your body gets all of the nutrients needed.

Becoming overwhelmed with the vegan learning curve

OVERCOME! It's OK, be gentle with yourself and the process. Don't expect perfection right away. The more you learn about being vegan, the quicker you'll learn how to cook dishes including some old favorites like mac 'n' cheese. You CAN do this, keep moving forward!

Depending on your current eating habits, your body goes through a detox phase with potentially unpleasant symptoms.

OVERCOME! Realize that this is a possible reaction, especially if you have been eating a lot of animal products and processed foods. Listen to your body and give it time to heal. Be sure that you are eating a variety of fruits, vegetables, grains and proteins. You may feel that a vegan diet will not work for you when really all you may need is to make more gradual changes.

Transitional Vegan

This is the route I chose to go. So after I had my "a-ha" moment to become vegan I knew it wouldn't be easy but I also knew that I could do it at my pace. I decided to become vegetarian first. I was vegetarian for three months before becoming full-blown vegan. I cleaned out my pantry, fridge and freezer of all animal products. The only non-vegan food that remained in my freezer was dairy ice cream. I chose to become vegetarian first because I still enjoyed eating sushi and ice cream.

It was pretty easy for me to remove meat from my diet but I felt like I had to start all over with my cooking skills. I knew how to cook meat in a healthy way and make it the star but I did not know how to do the same for vegetables. I started buying faux meat products and found them to be disgusting and bogged me down so I did some research on how to cook vegan healthfully and with whole, real foods.

During my research I came across this badass blog, Ohsheglows.com. Angela's inspirational writing and to die for recipes inspired me to try new foods and cooking techniques. I continued to work out about 5 times a week at the same intensity but I was not fueling my body with enough calories. I lost 10-15 pounds. Now you may think, yes, that is awesome! Well, it would have been if I had 10-15 pounds to spare. Unfortunately, that was not the case. I am a petite chick who was burning through my fuel faster than I could replenish it. So I had the "difficult" task of eating!! I am in love with the fact that the way I gained weight was to add in nuts, avocados, larger portions, more protein and complex carbs and a variety of fruits and veggies.

Before making my transition I was suckered into marketing schemes and terms such as "low fat," "fat free," "sugar free," etc.

What they don't tell you is that when they take something like fat or sugar out of a product they replace it with an evil cocktail of chemicals to try and make that product taste good. Anyways, at first when I lost that weight I felt weak, sure, you could see my abs and every muscle in my body was cut, but I felt lethargic. I have always been proud of the fact that I am a small chick with junk in the trunk. Well I lost my junk, not cool. Once I found my body's perfect balance of exercise and food intake I feel stronger than I ever have, I have lasting energy, my skin is clear, and I feel awesome!

Not only am I experiencing physical advantages, I also experienced a beautiful mental shift. I feel more at peace with myself knowing that what I eat, wear and put on my body is not harming any other creature. In fact, now that I feel more at peace I am most certainly more happy, which is key to a fulfilling life.

Going back now to eliminating ice cream and fish from my diet. Since I was in fact detoxing my body from animal products I became more sensitive to fish. A couple of times while I was vegetarian I ate fish but became queasy each time. It wasn't too difficult for me to get rid of fish because there are tasty veggie sushi options. Ice cream was the last thing containing animal products that I removed from my diet. Ice cream was last because it was more of an emotional crutch for me. Growing up, if someone wanted to cheer me up they would take me out for ice cream. After learning techniques to deal with my emotions such as yoga and hiking I was able to let go of ice cream for good. Besides, I enjoy the taste of coconut ice cream 1,000,000 times more than traditional ice cream.

Advantages

You give your body time to get used to eating clean, fresh, whole plant foods.

Less likely to experience extreme detox effects.

Give yourself time to mentally prepare for what being vegan will be like.

In my experience, more likely to succeed on a vegan diet.

You will lose weight, maybe not as quick as someone cold turkey, but that also depends on what you choose to keep in your diet. If you choose to keep cheese in your diet you will lose weight slower than choosing to keep fish in your diet.

Challenges

Not sure where to start with preparing meals.

OVERCOME! Have a variety of vegan blogs, books, videos and magazines with excellent, simple to make food. All of my recipes are designed with the new vegan in mind using ingredients you likely already have in your kitchen.

Not losing weight.

OVERCOME! Many times people become vegetarian before vegan, which is all good, but many of them end up relying too much on cheese and other dairy products, actually causing them to gain weight. If you choose the transitional path I recommend only consuming a very minimal amount of dairy in a week. Studies have shown cheese to be addicting, which is why many people feel they can't give it up.

Don't know what to order at restaurants.

OVERCOME! There are excellent resources all over the web about vegan-friendly restaurants. If for whatever reason you can't find a menu online of the restaurant you are going to stick to my guidelines in chapter 5.

Not getting enough nutrients your body needs especially if active.

OVERCOME! Research is critical in changing your lifestyle. I recommend getting your blood work done to see where you may be lacking nutrients. Once you find out the results I have an entire chapter dedicated to getting the essential nutrients such as B12, calcium and iron into your diet.

Tips for a successful transition

Stock Your Pantry

I find this to be absolutely crucial! Even before becoming vegan I had a rule in my house—in order to keep temptation at bay do not have it in the house! Of course, there are times when I enjoy indulgences, normally ice cream. Like having the right tools to do the job and having the right stock items in your pantry make your transition much easier.

So what's in my pantry? I have a variety of beans such as black beans, cannellini beans, garbanzo beans, kidney beans and pinto beans. Variety of grains such as millet, quinoa, spelt berries, wheat berries, amaranth, brown rice, steel cut oats and rolled oats. Flours for baking; I always have all-purpose unbleached flour, spelt flour, garbanzo flour, oat flour, whole wheat flour and whole wheat pastry flour.

I also have a little something sweet, all unrefined sweeteners; raw organic sugar, brown sugar, coconut sugar, blackstrap molasses, brown rice syrup and agave. Variety of nut, seeds and nut butters such as hemp seeds, pepitas, pistachios, almonds, cashews, walnuts, pecans, sunflower seeds. Last but not least I have a variety of spices such as nutritional yeast, cumin, coriander, allspice, paprika, turmeric, cayenne pepper,

Italian spice blend and curry powders.

Research

Something I found very helpful is to do your homework...like you are doing right now! By reading vegan books, vegan cookbooks, checking out vegan blogs and vegan Youtube channels. I also believe it is important to research what type of struggles vegans experience with meeting dietary needs. The major ones I found cause problems are deficiency in iron, vitamin B12, protein, and calcium. My go-to source for iron are dark leafy greens, broccoli, beans, lentils, whole grains and blackstrap molasses. My favorite and primary source for vitamin B12 is nutritional yeast; I sprinkle this nutty cheesy powder from heaven on everything!

I get my protein from basically the same places as my iron—beans, lentils, tempeh, tofu, whole grains, nuts and seeds. Calcium seems to really stump people when transitioning to veganism, as the dairy industry brainwashes us that you can only get calcium from cow's milk. Well, well, where do you think cows get their calcium from—the food they eat, grass. I get my calcium from dark leafy greens, beans, tofu, soy and almond milk.

Focus on What You Add, Not Take Away

I think this is the main reason I felt like I had to start all over when learning how to cook vegan. I focused so much on the fact that certain items were now out of my diet, how could I possibly survive?! Ha, well turns out I was missing the fact that I literally have hundreds of "new" foods available to try, experiment with and have fun with!

Some foods I eat now that I never did when I ate meat: butternut squash, kombucha squash, pumpkin, fennel, pomegranate, patty pan squash, eggplant, hummus, pinto beans, quinoa, wheatberries, hemp seeds, chia seeds, kale, rainbow chard, tempeh and so many more!

This is supposed to be fun! Get in the kitchen, put on some tunes, grab a new recipe and get after it!

Be Prepared

As the Boy Scouts would say, be prepared! They are right. I find having a grocery list of what you are preparing to eat for the week and the ingredients you need to purchase keeps me on track to purchase only what I need for the week and not buy packaged vegan foods. If you are strapped for time during the week, try making large batches of beans and grains so you can easily throw your meals for the week together. When going out, I recommend looking at the menu ahead of time to know if there is something you can eat. If you don't see anything you can always call the restaurant ahead of time to see if the chef can prepare something for you. Believe it or not, chefs are very happy to make something special and vegan for you; it gives them a chance to be creative and do something out of the ordinary.

Go Easy on Yourself

Making the transition to a vegan diet is one of the most compassionate decisions you can make for animals around the world. Sometimes we forget how to be compassionate with other humans, especially ourselves. Know that becoming vegan is truly a journey, whether you get there cold turkey or by becoming vegetarian first. There is no wrong way to become vegan and it is a unique process for each person, as long as you keep moving forward with your decision and know that this is the best thing for your health and the welfare of animals.

Trust me, there have been a few times I ate a piece of bread only to find out afterwards it had an egg wash on it. There was one time I had a piece of bread that contained butter, egg and milk! Well, crap! That is the first thing I remember saying to myself after eating that. Afterwards, I decided to learn from the experience instead of beat myself up. I just need to remember next time to ask if there is any egg or dairy in the bread. These questions will become second nature eventually.

Telling Friends and Family

Telling my friends and family was interesting. Before I decided to become vegan, my brother had already started his vegan journey four years prior. He and I approached veganism in different ways. He approached it from a health and religious standpoint where I approached it from an ethical stand. Either way is great; like I said, there is no wrong way to become vegan. For the most part my friends and family were supportive; they just worried about my wilting away and blowing away with the breeze.

I showed them! If I wilted away I wouldn't have been able to compete in numerous races, rock climb, do mud runs, snowboarding, and oh so much more! And YOU will show all of the doubters out there too!

Once becoming vegan and you tell strangers/acquaintances your dietary choice you will notice that suddenly they are health and nutrition experts and know what is best for you. For those types of people the best way to speak with them is through facts and knowledge about the foods you eat and where you get your protein, calcium, iron, etc. Other people are genuinely concerned with your well-being and just want you to be healthy. You can swamp them with facts but really explain to them the reason(s) you chose to become vegan, it is important to you. If they love you, they will understand and respect your decision.

Vegan Impact on the World

There is an assortment of reasons to become vegan but typically a person has one specific reason why they want to become vegan. The three most common reasons are for health, the environment and the ethical treatment of animals. My personal journey to veganism started because of the ethical treatment of animals. Although I became vegan for the animals, I had no idea how becoming vegan helps improve the health of my body and the environment as well.

Go Vegan for YOUR Health

This portion of the book is jam-packed with facts. So bear with me while I knowledge dump on you, as this information may save your life or the life of someone you know! Let's jump in! Vegan diets are generally lower in total fat, saturated fats, HDL cholesterol (bad cholesterol) than non-vegan diets. Many studies have shown that vegan diets lower your risk of coronary disease, diabetes, and some forms of cancers. Not only do vegan diets benefit you in this way, but you will likely experience an increase in sustained energy, and weight loss.

Lower Your Risk of Chronic Diseases

Cancer

Vegans tend to have a lower chance of getting cancer than both meat eaters AND vegetarians. A whopping 34% lower chance of female-specific cancers such as breast and ovarian cancer. Eating a vegan diet removes the cancer-promoting growth hormone IGF-1 whereas animal foods actually promote the production of this hormone. On another note, what you choose to eat can actually change your genes. So even if you have a history of cancer or any chronic disease in your family you do have the choice and control to change them just by what you put on your plate. Pretty powerful stuff, eh?

A healthful plant diet can reverse cardiovascular damage. Don't believe me? During a study at the Cleveland Clinic, they cured 18 patients with established coronary disease with a whole-food, plant-based diet. Not only did the diet stop the progression of the disease but 70% of patients experienced a reversal of blocked arteries.

With higher cholesterol levels there is also an increased risk of heart attack. Each point cholesterol goes up you have a 2% greater risk of having a heart attack. Reversely is the same though! For each point lowered in cholesterol you have a 2% decrease likelihood of heart attack. The average American's cholesterol is 210 while the average vegetarian's cholesterol is 161—that is a huge margin! The foods that vegans eat are naturally free of cholesterol helping to drastically reduce the risk of heart attack.

Heart attack. Doesn't it seem like everyone around you is developing some form of heart health problem? It's so sad because it is a completely preventable disease with a healthy diet. Luckily there is good news: cardiovascular disease can be defeated with a vegan diet! In a controlled study funded by the Physicians Committee for Responsible Medicine studied a group of 99 participants in Washington D.C. for 22 weeks; the participants followed a low-fat, low-glycemic vegan diet or guidelines prescribed by the ADA. Note that all of the participants had type 2 diabetes.

The vegan group improved significantly in every Alternative Healthy Eating Index category; the higher the AHEI score, the lower the risk of cardiovascular disease. The vegan group increased intake of vegetables, fruits, nut and soy protein, and cereal fiber, and a decrease in trans-fat intake.

Both groups were able to reduce their weight and their hemoglobin A1c, a measure of blood sugar levels over a prolonged period of time. However, the vegan group experienced more significant reductions in both categories.

"The results of this study suggest that, if followed for the long-term, a low-fat vegan diet may be associated with a reduced risk of major chronic diseases, particularly cardiovascular disease," the study concludes.

Arthritis

Arthritis really just means inflammation of a joint. Vegan diets are naturally low in inflammation-causing foods. Some of the top food offenders that promote inflammation are animal fats, simple carbohydrates such as white bread, and refined sugars (white sugar). Some foods that reduce inflammation in the body are whole grains, dark leafy greens, nuts especially walnuts and almonds, cherries and bright bell peppers just to name a few. After a day of strenuous workout or if my knee feels a little funny I am sure to enjoy plenty of cherries to fight inflammation.

Lasting Energy All Day

Have you ever experienced the dreaded afternoon slump? You know, you're going through your work day and notice it's about 2:00 pm and you feel exhausted? You head to the break room for a cup of coffee to perk up only to not be able to sleep that night? I sure remember those days! Many people find that when transitioning to a vegan diet they experience an increased amount of energy during physical activity and don't experience the mid-afternoon crash.

From personal experience the only reason I felt a lack of energy is because I was not eating enough food for the amount of activity I was doing. Once I found that "sweet spot" of activity-to-food ratio I experienced energy all day. I truly believe that you are what you eat so I like to fuel my body with either a green smoothie or a big bowl of oats first thing in the morning.

A substantial breakfast helps keep you full through the morning until lunch. I know that if I fueled my body with a box of vegan cookies in the morning instead of my glorious smoothie, I would be hungry in about an hour and feel sluggish all day. This is why I stress so much to eat whole foods instead of relying on so-called energy bars and packaged foods for meals. Don't get me wrong, in a pinch I will reach for a vegan energy bar, but trust me, your body will LOVE the real plant foods you feed it.

Weight Loss

Another thoughtful reason people adopt a vegan lifestyle is to lose weight. However, once the weight is off some people fall back into their previous eating habits and gain the weight back. First of all, making the switch to a vegan diet is a lifestyle change, not a fad diet. You will more than likely lose weight because you will greatly reduce or even eliminate all animal products right away which are full of artery clogging, fat promoting animal fats. When these leave your diet you will lose weight. Also, since I do not condone processed foods you will lose weight because those things are just jam-packed full of artificial sweeteners, trans fats and artificial colors just to list a few. When these are removed from your diet your body will naturally detoxify itself.

Wow, right?! I had no idea that eating a healthy vegan diet could impact health in this way, and keep in mind, this is only a limited list of health benefits. All right, so our health is now in check, but what about the health of the earth? Keep on reading to learn how your new vegan lifestyle is improving the health of our planet.

Go Vegan for the Environment

Before becoming vegan, I had no idea how eating meat negatively impacted the environment in a variety of ways. If every person swapped just one meat meal a week for a vegan meal, these numbers would drastically decrease. We only have one earth, people, it's not like we have a Plan B.

Save the Rainforest

Take a moment and imagine the sounds of a waterfall intertwined by the magical sound of tropical birds. Feel the warm mist of the jungle floor on your skin and the smell of tropical flowers blooming. Now imagine the smell of cow dung and the sound of frightened animals. That is exactly what is happening to the earth's rainforests.

Every second of every day, a football-size space of the rainforest is destroyed to make space to raise livestock. The animals raised here are slaughtered and shipped to the United States to be sold as cheap fast food burgers. With each square foot of rainforest that is destroyed roughly 30 plant species, 100 different insects, and dozens of birds, mammals and reptiles are destroyed.

Depleting Natural Resources

Water: There are more than 17 BILLION livestock animals round the world, which is triple the amount of people on the earth. It sure does take a lot of water to keep these animals alive. It takes 2,464 gallons of water to produce just one pound of beef. To put that number into perspective that is the same as if you took a seven-minute shower every day for 6 months. On the flip side, it only takes 25 gallons of water to grow one pound of wheat.

Topsoil: The major grains used to feed livestock are soybeans and corn, which causes massive erosion. It is estimated that we lose nearly 7 billion tons of topsoil every year. PETA reports "of all agriculture land in the United States, 87% is used to raise animals for food. That's 45% of the total land mass in the US. About 260 million acres of US forest have been cleared to create cropland to produce feed for animals raised for food. The meat industry is directly responsible for 85% of all soil erosion in the United States."

Fossil Fuels: Animal agriculture uses 10% of the energy used in the United States every year. "Producing just one hamburger uses enough fuel to drive a small car 20 miles. Of all raw materials and fossil fuels used in the US, more than 1/3 is devoted to raising animals for food."

Stinky Situation

Dear citizens of earth, the earth is warming because of a variety of different reasons. Be sure to turn off your lights when not in use, carpool, ride your bike, walk, buy an electric car, recycle. What the government doesn't tell you is that emissions from factory farms contribute to toxic greenhouse gases more than all of the trucks and cars on the planet! Animal crap releases methane and nitrous oxide, which are two highly potent greenhouse gasses. Choosing to replace even just one meat meal a week with a vegan meal can significantly help these numbers; imagine what cutting out animals altogether can do??!

Agriculture Run-Off

Keeping with the poop talk, livestock produces 87,000 pound of poop per second! Holy crap! In factory farms the animals' urine and feces are funneled into a lagoon where many times it breaks and gets to our streams, rivers and lakes that we get our drinking water from. These waste lagoons also emit dangerous gases; ammonia, hydrogen sulfide and methane.

People who live around these factory farms breathe in these gases, causing irreversible damage to their health such as sore throats, seizures and shortness of breath. Drinking contaminated water causes other health problems such as blue baby syndrome which causes death in infants and unexpected abortions. On top of all that, since the majority of factory farms give their animals antibiotics for growth these also get into our water system which we drink and make it more difficult to combat human illnesses.

"A typical pig factory generates the same amount of raw waste as a city of 12,000 people. According to the Environmental Protection Agency, raising animals for food is the number-one source of water pollution."

"More than 80 percent of the corn we grow and more than 95 percent of the oats are fed to livestock. The world's cattle alone consume a quantity of food equal to the caloric needs of 8.7 billion people—more than the entire human population on Earth. According to the Worldwatch Institute, "Roughly 2 of every 5 tons of grain produced in the world is fed to livestock, poultry, or fish; decreasing consumption of these products, especially of beef, could free up massive quantities of grain and reduce pressure on land."

Isn't it amazing how what we choose to put on our plates can drastically improve the health of the environment that we all share? Remember, we only have one place to live; there is no Plan B. Now for the animals, people as a whole feel that animal abuse is wrong. What many do not realize is that factory farmed animals are abused every day. They are abused either by their terrible living conditions or by the people who handle them. It's time for people to make the connection where their food really comes from.

Go Vegan for the Animals

I am what you call an ethical vegan. All that really means is that I do not eat meat or animal products because I do not want to contribute to the suffering of any creature. In the back of my mind I always knew that the business of killing animals for meat was an ugly one, I just chose to ignore the facts so I could continue to eat steaks and chicken breasts. When I decided to open my mind and my heart to what injustices these animals faced that was a game changer. In the following paragraphs I provide information on these animals' living conditions, since they are horrendous enough without adding the cruelty and abuse they experience from the workers.

Animals Used for Food

Broiler Chickens: Each year in just the United States 9 billion chickens are killed. They are "raised" in huge ammonia-filled windowless sheds with artificial lighting forcing them to eat continuously. Once they are large enough they are sent to slaughter where they are hung upside down by their feet, throats slit by machines and dumped into scalding water to de-feather them.

Egg Laying Chickens: Most of these creatures spend their entire life in a battery cage stacked upon each other in a giant warehouse. These cages do not allow for the chickens to even spread their wings; because of this the chickens experience feather loss, skin chafes and crippled feet. Once the chicks are hatched they are sorted between males and females; the females continue down the line to later have the same life as their mother while the male chicks deemed worthless in the egg industry are thrown into a grinding machine ALIVE!

Pigs: Pigs have a cognitive ability higher than dogs and three-year-old children. They are very social and playful animals and form very strong social bonds. Unfortunately, pigs in factory farms spend most of their life in a gestation cage which are 7 feet long and 2 feet wide, not enough space to even turn around.

Picture for a minute, you are flying cross-country, you head back to coach, you strap in. There you are this is your seat for the next few hours. Well, if you are anything like me you need to get up, move around and stretch. What if you got into that seat, buckled in and were told you could not get out of that seat for the rest of your life. That is the life of a pig in a gestation cage.

A sow is artificially inseminated many times in her life where she gives birth and her babies are taken from her in 10 days. Then the process starts over again until the sow's body is so worn she is sent to slaughter. Wonder what happens to the piglets that were taken from their mom? They are confined in pens, the males are castrated without painkillers. These conditions are very crowded and the pigs are driven to destructive behaviors such as cannibalism and tail biting. So farmers chop off the pigs' tails and break their teeth off all without the use of painkillers.

Cows: Dairy cows are treated like milk-pumping machines instead of intelligent, emotional creatures. A dairy cow is artificially inseminated shortly after her first birthday, gives birth, has her baby ripped away from her almost immediately and is pumped by cold machines for 10 months while she lactates. Once she is done lactating the insemination process starts again.

Some cows spend their entire lives standing on cold concrete floors living in their own waste. Once the baby is one day old it is taken away in a cart and chained to a pen. The calf spends its life lying down and fed a diet low in iron to keep the skin pale for the veal market.

Did you ever wonder why some people feel they are addicted or dependent upon milk? Casein, a protein found in all mammal milk including human, when digested releases opiates into the brain helping the mother and baby bonding experience. These animals are also pumped with antibiotics and growth hormones which in turn humans drink.

While you're thinking, also ponder this, humans are the only animal that drink milk after infancy and the only animal that drinks the milk of another species. You wouldn't see a giraffe drinking milk from a rhino, would you?! Dairy is the number one food allergy among infants...hmmm, I wonder why!

Turkeys: 248 million turkeys are raised and slaughtered each year; 77 million are consumed during Thanksgiving, Christmas and Easter. Prior to being killed these intelligent birds spend 5-6 months confined in cages in dark warehouses where they are de-beaked and toes cut without painkillers.

They are genetically manipulated to build large muscle. Because of this their internal organs are smooshed together and actually die because of it. Like their feathered friends the chicken, they are hung upside down by their brittle legs, heads dunked in an electric bath to stun them, they are still conscious, throats slit and dunked into scalding baths for de-feathering; many of these birds still alive when entering the de-feather tank.

Ducks and Geese: I have very fond memories of going to the park as a kid and feeding the ducks and geese and admiring how gracefully they swim. Did you know that ducks live in couples or groups and geese mate for life and mourn for long periods of time when its mate dies? Sadly for factory farmed ducks and geese they are crammed into tiny cages in where else, but dark warehouses. Ducks and geese that are raised for foie gras have pipes or tubes shoved down their throats three times a day so that four pounds of grain can be forced into their stomach develop the "fatty liver" that is foie gras. When their disease ridden livers are 10x their normal size they are sent to slaughter. That fancy liver still sound appetizing?

Fish and Shellfish: Despite what you may have heard, fish are intelligent and have the same pain response that birds and mammals experience. Sadly the fish industry kills nearly 6 billion fish each year and 245 animals are killed for sport. This industry is one of the least regulated industries, with the fish suffocated, crushed and gutted while fully conscious.

Personally, I do not feel an intense emotional connection to fish and shellfish; however, I do know the impact that commercial fishing has on the oceans. Not only are fish caught in gigantic nets but hundreds of sea turtles, dolphins, whales, and sea birds are caught in the traps, suffering and dying.

Animals for Clothing and Accessories

Leather: Leather can come from a variety of different animals, from cows to pigs, kangaroo to alligator. Leather directly supports factory farming. Many times when these animals are dismembered and skinned they are still conscious. Now, I get it, you look in your closet and your shoes, purses and belts are made of leather. Well, crap, right? No. Remember this is a journey, as you need to buy new clothes or belts buy products not made from animals. When it is time to do some spring cleaning consider donating your leather clothing items. This is a process and it is OK if it takes time to update your wardrobe.

Wool: Mary had a little lamb... cute song, right? Too bad a sheep's life nowadays isn't fun and frolicking like it should be. Instead, these gentle creatures live a life of fear.

Under normal circumstances a sheep will produce enough fleece to protect itself but with genetic modification these sheep produce way more than needed. Shearers get paid by volume instead of by the hour so shearing is fast and sloppy oftentimes shearing off chunks of skin and even shearing off half of a sheep's face.

Fur: Furs come from one or two places, either a creature from the wild or animals from fur farms. Either way these animals suffered and had a terrible death. Animals on fur farms spend their entire lives in tiny wire cages. Fur farming uses extremely cruel methods of killing such as suffocation, electrocution, gas and poisoning. About half of the fur in the U.S. comes from China where dogs and cats experience tremendous pain and are deliberately mislabeled when the furs come to the states.

Animals that are trapped in the wild are caught with a steel leg clamp where the animal is left there for days to suffer from blood loss, shock, dehydration and attacks from predators. Conibear traps capture the animals around the necks with 90 pounds of pressure per square inch. Water-set traps capture beavers causing the animals to struggle for roughly nine minutes before they drown.

So yes, this is all freaking awful and cruel. The good news is that there are a huge number of cruelty-free fabrics that are just as stylish and warm that you can feel good knowing no creature suffered for fashion. If you want my honest opinion I think that fur looks pretentious.

Animal Testing: Cosmetics and Cleaning Supplies

The United States is really behind the times in animal testing of cosmetics. Rabbits are confined with a metal clamp around their necks so they cannot move their heads when companies such as Johnson & Johnson drop a particular liquid in the rabbit's eye to see how long it takes for the cornea to burn.

These methods are cruel and inhumane, especially now that there are ways to test products without testing them on animals. As you begin to read labels you will notice the companies that do not test on animals also do not contain cancerous ingredients such as parabens, fragrance, silicone and more.

Cruelty Free Cosmetics

The FDA constitutes a cosmetic as "skin moisturizers, perfumes, lipsticks, fingernail polishes, eye and facial makeup preparations, cleansing shampoos, permanent waves, hair colors, and deodorants, as well as any substance intended for use as a component of a cosmetic product."

Cosmetics

Drug Store Brands

Almay

NYX

E.L.F. aka Eyes Lips Face

Hard Candy

Physician's Formula

High End Store Brands

Smashbox

Bobbi Brown

Urban Decay

Juice Beauty by Alicia Silverstone

Too Faced Cosmetics

M.A.C.

Stila

Body Products

Dr. Bronner's Magic Soaps

Kiss my Face

Toms of Maine

Jasons

Alba Botanica

All Purpose Cleaning Supplies

Seventh Generation (can be found in large supermarkets)

EO Products

Method cleaning products

Mrs. Meyers Clean Day products

OrganiWorks

How to Be a Healthy Vegan

Before we jump into what being a healthy vegan means I want you to know that you do not have to be perfect and fit this mold. The longer you are vegan the more you will discover which includes vegan junk food. There are some delectable vegan cookies, raw cheesecakes, brownies, ice cream, chips even cookie dough! I am all about once in a while indulgences because without them culinary life would be dull. For the majority of time, though, it is important to eat a well-rounded whole foods diet. That way when you do indulge it won't be the end of the world. So let's jump in!

Tinya's Vegan Story

Because my mother was an animal rights activist in the 1970s, I was raised vegetarian for compassion reasons. I remember we ate a significant amount of cheese, and a glass of milk accompanied each and every dinner. I started struggling with my weight in middle school, as it always amazed people I was a "dieting" vegetarian. By the mid 1990s I learned that the meat and dairy industries had strong connections. It was shocking to discover the direct correlations between diary and veal. So began my journey to a vegan lifestyle. I did not find it easy in the beginning. In fact, it took my husband and me nearly 7 years to transition from vegetarian to vegan; ditching milk first, then cheese, with eggs being the very last to be let go.

Once I fully embraced veganism, the transformation was not only physical, but also very psychological. For the first time, I didn't need to "diet," while naturally maintaining a comfortable and healthy size. I felt a complete sense of peace, becoming more confident than ever about my food choices. I have since had two vegan pregnancies with zero complications; both babies born at above average weights.

My husband, also vegan, is a firefighter and in the best shape of his life at the age of 42. As a family, we thrive on health and consciousness, while never looking back to our egg and dairy days.

Eat a Well-Rounded Vegan Diet

What you choose to eat can either heal you or harm you. Food has an amazing ability to heal you physically and mentally. I have a mantra that I say to myself every day to make sure I eat a wide variety of foods. "Eat the color of the rainbow with a sprinkle of nuts, beans and grains." When you eat a variety of colors you are also eating a variety of essential vitamins and minerals. Fruits and veggies typically fall under these colors: red, orange, yellow, white, tan/brown, green, purple and blue.

Green! Are you sick of me talking about dark leafy greens yet? No? That's good because I cannot say enough good things about green fruits and veggies. It is a goal of mine every day to eat dark leafy greens in one way or another. Green vegetables are good for your eyes, bones and teeth, and their vitamin K content helps your blood to clot properly. These foods' antioxidant vitamins, particularly vitamins C and E, may lower your risk of chronic diseases. Oh man, the list for greens I love is huge, get ready now! Artichokes, arugula, spinach, kale, rainbow chard, asparagus, broccoli, cabbage, zucchini, kiwi, green grapes, peas, green onion, just to name a few.

Purple and blue fruits and veggies are just beautiful. Blueberries are definitely in my top three favorite fruits. So cute and tiny and exploding with sweet juicy yumminess! Not only do they taste outstanding, blue and purple fruits are also full of anthocyanins, natural plant pigments with powerful antioxidant properties that may reduce your risk of cardiovascular disease. They also contain flavonoids and ellagic acid, compounds that may destroy cancer cells. In my opinion these are the most beautiful fruits and veggies, the blue and purple variety. I love eggplant, blackberries, blueberries, acai berry, purple potatoes, purple cabbage, plums, pomegranates, elderberry and more.

Red fruits and veggies are loaded with antioxidants including lycopene and anthocyanins which fight heart disease and prostate cancer. Some of my favorite red produce are strawberries, raspberries, cranberries, cherries, beets, red bell pepper, blood oranges, red onions, red grapes and many more.

Orange/yellow fruits and veggies are packed with zeaxanthin, flavonoids, lycopene, potassium, vitamin C and beta-carotene, which is vitamin A helping you be a badass every day. My favorite orange and yellow fruits and veggies are butternut squash, cantaloupe, carrots, mangos, peaches, sweet potatoes, pumpkin, sweet corn, yellow squash, yellow pears and more!

White fruits and veggies are the internal scrubbers. You know those sucker fish that you put in the fish tank to clean it? That's what I imagine white produce is doing for my inners. White fruits and veggies are high in dietary fiber, helping to protect you from high cholesterol, and antioxidant-rich flavonoids, such as quercetin, which is abundant in apples and pears. My favorite white fruits and veggies are bananas, dates, ginger, garlic, turnips, parsnips, cauliflower and more!

The Essential Vegan

Green	**Purple/Blue**	**Red/Pink**	**Orange/Yellow**	**White**
Artichokes	Currants	Beets	Apricots	Bananas
Arugula	Blackberries	Blood oranges	Butternut squash	Pears
Asparagus	Blueberries	Red bell pepper	Sweet potatoes	Cauliflower
Avocados	Plums	Cranberries	Oranges	Garlic
Broccoli	Eggplant	Papaya	Lemons	Ginger
Kale	Elderberry	Raspberries	Cantaloupe	Jicama
Celery	Purple grapes	Radishes	Carrots	Mushrooms
Cabbage	Pomegranates	Red apples	Mangoes	Onions
Cucumbers	Prunes	Red onions	Yellow squash	Parsnips
Endive	Purple cabbage	Red potatoes	Pumpkin	Potatoes
Grapes	Purple potatoes	Strawberries	Pineapple	Shallots
Peppers	Purple carrots	Tomatoes	Peaches	Turnips
Honeydew	Figs	Watermelon	Sweet corn	Peaches
Kiwi	Raisins	Grapefruit	Yellow beets	Nectarines
Lettuce	Acai berry	Pomegranates	Acorn squash	Asparagus
Leeks	Purple Asparagus	Cherries	Permissions	Daikon radish
Lime	Purple Peppers	Rhubarb	Kumquats	White corn
Peas				
Snow peas				
Spinach				
Watercress				
Zucchini				
Swiss chard				
Brussels Sprouts				

Get Your Blood Work Checked

I like to get my blood work checked once a year at my physical. I recommend going a couple months after you become vegan to gauge if you are lacking in nutrients. A typical blood test does not check for iron, calcium or vitamin B12 so you will need to ask for these to also be tested. It is critical to have your blood work tested to be sure that you are meeting the minimum requirements and your body is functioning properly. One fun thing to check is your cholesterol and watch it drop the longer you are vegan. Be sure to have the following tested: iron, calcium, B12, vitamin D and folate.

How to Receive Essential Nutrients from Food

Through a well-rounded vegan diet my body is able to get all of my vitamins, minerals and proteins from plants. The most common nutrients that are lacking in a vegan diet, especially a new vegan diet, are Vitamin B12, iron, calcium and vitamin D. Something interesting is that the general public is deficient in iron, calcium and vitamin D. Vegans tend to get a bad rap about a lack of nutrients because it is unfamiliar.

Vitamin B12: Vitamin B12 is essential to humans because it is responsible for cell division and blood production. This is especially important for pregnant and breastfeeding women and infants. Vitamin B12 comes from bacteria and animals ingest these bacteria which is how it gets into their bodies. Most people, though, do not produce enough B12 on their own. The primary source of B12 in American diets is from animal meat since all animals produce B12. Vegans need to be sure to incorporate B12-fortified foods into their diet. The most popular way is through nutritional yeast, which is an ingredient used in vegan cooking, or you can also purchase B12-fortified soy milk. I get my B12 from nutritional yeast by just sprinkling on a tablespoon on top of salads and in soups and sauces.

Iron: Iron is important in a human diet because it is a central part of hemoglobin which carries oxygen to the blood. Something important to note about iron is that you also should consume a fruit or veggie high in vitamin C to help the absorption of iron. My favorite ways to incorporate iron into my diet is through dark leafy greens, beans and tempeh. The highest sources of iron in plant foods are soybeans at 8.8 in 1 cup, blackstrap molasses 7.2mg in 2Tbs and lentils at 6.6mg in 1 cup.

Calcium: How many of us have been brainwashed into thinking that the best source of calcium comes from dairy? I know I sure was!! Man, I remember my mom would not let me leave the dinner table until I finished my glass of milk. I hated that. Calcium is important because it helps keep our bones strong and firm. Some excellent sources of plant-based calcium include cooked dark leafy greens including kale, bok choy, collard greens and more. More sources include beans, and soy products such as soybeans, tofu and tempeh.

Importance of Omega-3 Fatty Acids

Study after study show that omega-3s are essential for proper bodily and neurological development and function. Those who consume omega-3s have lower levels of depression, reduced inflammation in the body, improve memory and slow the process of Alzheimer's and dementia.

There are two types of omega-3 fatty acids; EPA/DHA primarily found in fish and ALA primarily found in plant foods such as nuts and seeds. Uh-oh, so I can only get EPA and DHA from fish? Lucky for us the fish are able to get these essential fatty acids from the algae they eat. So, my suggestion is to take a supplement of algae oil to receive your EPA and DHA omega-3s. The ALA omega-3s are much easier for us to find. The top sources for plant based omegs-3s are chia seeds, flax seed – be sure it is ground and hemp seeds. While other nuts and seeds such as walnuts are wonderful for our health, they are not as dense in omega-3s as the hemp, chia and flax seeds.

When Food Just Isn't Enough, Supplement

Personally, I do not feel the need to supplement my diet with nutrients in other forms besides food. However, if you get your blood work back and find you need to supplement that's OK. Just be sure to take the right supplements from reputable companies with high standards. The FDA does not regulate what goes into supplements so much of what is on the market right now is not even really helping you. The most common supplements vegans need are B12, Vitamin D, Iron and Calcium. Some of the top natural brands are NOW, Solgar, and Vitamin Code. Please be sure to consult your doctor before starting supplementation to your diet.

Will I Get Sick Less on a Vegan Diet?

Just because you become vegan does not mean that you are totally immune to any nasty virus that comes our way. What it DOES mean, though, is that we are sick a lot less and for a shorter duration. Pre-vegan I could count on getting sick once during the winter and once in the spring. My winter illness was typically due to something along the lines of a wicked cold or cough that would turn into an ear infection and could last for 2 weeks to a month. I would get all drugged up on antibiotics but never really cure myself. In the spring I would experience terrible sinus infections that would cause my face to feel like a faucet, my nose would be running constantly and I couldn't control, sexy image, eh?

After becoming vegan and conducting research on food and health, I learned that food can keep your immune system strong, combating nasty bacteria and viruses that so many of us experience. Since becoming vegan, when the rest of the world around me is getting the flu, coughs and colds, I am drinking and eating the colors of the rainbow helping me combat all that crap.

Since becoming vegan almost three years ago I did get a sinus infection once and it lasted 5 days instead of weeks and weeks. Not only do highly nutrient dense foods keep our bodies strong but so do herbs! I had no clue that certain herbs and spices have antiviral and antibacterial properties. During the cold and flu season I am sure to incorporate certain foods into my diet every day. Raw citrus such as oranges and lemons are high in vitamin C and flavonoids which boosts white blood cells and immune system.

Favorite Sickness Fighting Herbs!

Garlic: Raw garlic is also another exceptional food to incorporate into your diet. Does raw garlic sound too extreme for ya? I thought so too; the only way I incorporate raw garlic into my system is through juicing. Garlic is an herbal wonder drug containing antibacterial, antifungal and antiviral properties. Garlic also hinders free radicals from spreading in the body.

When preparing garlic for a recipe, after chopping or crushing, allow it sit at room temperature for 15 minutes before adding to the recipe. This triggers an enzyme reaction boosting the health compound in garlic.

Ginger: I absolutely fell in love with ginger incorporated into my juices. It provides a lovely warming sensation which helps blood circulation, reduces inflammation and supports the respiratory system. Drinking ginger tea or juice after eating aids in digestion. If you have a hurt stomach or even PMS pains, ladies, grate some ginger into your tea and enjoy the warming comfort.

Some ways to enjoy the healing benefits of ginger are through juicing, in tea form, making a ginger sweetener, ginger candy and in cooked foods such as stir-fry.

Turmeric: This beautiful herb looks a lot like fresh ginger, only orange instead of white inside. You can also readily find it in grocery stores ground. This herb is gaining a lot of popularity these days and for good reasons. Turmeric is like a medicine cabinet in one fabulous little package. It can aid in healing the following:

Aids in digestion and cleansing the liver

Lowering high blood pressure

Supports the immune system, protecting you from colds, flus and cough

Eases muscular and joint pain

Promotes healthy skin and heals skin

In order to get the most benefit from turmeric it is suggested that you take with some fresh ground black pepper. The black pepper improves the bioavailability of the turmeric, making smaller doses more available.

Cayenne pepper: This beautiful red spice is bursting with vitamin A, helping the body boost the immune system to fight illness, along with beta-carotene, vitamin E, vitamin C, calcium and potassium! Cayenne pepper is known to clean out the plaque from your arteries and also gets rid of LDL cholesterol. This pepper also has antifungal properties, so if you have any kind of fungal infection of the skin you can apply the spice directly on the affected area.

The best way to enjoy this spice is on food. Try putting it in a shaker and sprinkle it on all sorts of things from your morning tofu scramble to smoothies and juices.

Apple cider vinegar: Apple cider vinegar (ACV) is vinegar with a unique combination of vitamins, minerals and amino acids. Recent studies show that ACV helps lower glucose levels by 4-6%, which is great news for diabetics! ACV has also been shown to aid in weight loss by making people feel fuller longer. ACV aids in digestion; I would know. I drink 2 tsp every morning with a glass of water making for a nice, easy bathroom visit each morning. It is also excellent to use as a topical treatment for acne, warts and skin tags. I just dab a bit directly onto a problem area and leave on overnight. The next morning the skin problem is normally gone or at least significantly improved.

To get the most out of your apple cider vinegar mix it with either warm or cool water or juice. I like to enjoy 2Tbs mixed with 16 oz water, cinnamon, and sweetener.

Natural Home Remedies

Natural Cough Syrup

2 Tbs raw organic honey

2 Tbs Apple cider vinegar

2 Tbs water

¼ tsp cayenne pepper

¼ tsp cinnamon

Apple Cider Vinegar Drink

8-12 oz warm water

Juice of 1 lemon

2 tsp apple cider vinegar

1 tsp agave

Sprinkle of cayenne pepper

Note *only use warm water as hot water will pasteurize the vinegar therefore killing the beneficial enzymes.*

Immunity Boosting Juice

Ingredients:

2 large carrots

2 medium oranges with peel removed

1 large beet

1 cup cilantro

1 garlic clove

1 inch fresh ginger root

1/8 tsp cayenne pepper

Directions:

Chop fruits and vegetables into sizes able to fit in the juicer. Be sure to put fruits and veggies in at random so it mixes well. Once all is juiced sprinkle on the cayenne pepper for a boost of antiviral properties!

Now you have some recipes bursting with highly nutritious foods and herbs to battle any bad bugs that come your way! I want to expand a bit more about how a vegan diet can potentially improve heart health, prevent and reverse arthritis.

Vegan = Healthy Heart

Every part of our body is important but I have to say that the heart is at the top of my most important body parts. Without a healthy ticker life is very limited and not so fun. Dean Ornish, M.D., is the founder and president of the non-profit Preventive Medicine Research Institute, where he holds the Safeway Chair, and Clinical Professor of Medicine at the University of California, San Francisco.

For over 30 years, Dr. Ornish has directed clinical research demonstrating, for the first time, that comprehensive lifestyle changes may begin to reverse even severe coronary heart disease, without drugs or surgery.

Dean Ornish, MD, says that you absolutely can reverse at least some of the damage of even severe heart disease. "Our studies show that, with significant lifestyle changes, blood flow to the heart and its ability to pump normally improve in less than a month, and the frequency of chest pains fell by

90% in that time," Ornish says. "Within a year on our program, even severely blocked arteries in the heart became less blocked, and there was even more reversal after five years. That's compared with the natural history in other patients in our study, in which the heart just got worse and worse." In essence, that means becoming a vegetarian, filling your plate with fruits and vegetables, whole grains, legumes, soy products, nonfat dairy, and egg whites, and keeping away from fats, refined sugar, and carbohydrates. "You want to eat foods in their natural form as much as possible," Ornish says.

Prevent & Reverse Arthritis

Another rock star doctor is Joel Furhman, MD; he is a board-certified family physician, NEW YORK TIMES best-selling author and nutritional researcher who specializes in preventing and reversing disease through nutritional and natural methods. You can find interviews of Dr. Fuhrman from the *Dr. OZ show, The Today Show, Good Morning American and Live with Kelly.*

Now back to arthritis, the conventional cures for osteoarthritis and rheumatoid arthritis are either toxic drugs to reduce pain and inflammation and/or surgery. Every year, one million new cases are diagnosed and numbers are growing. Fortunately there is another treatment doctors like Dr. Furhman are starting to explore. Diet, specifically a vegan diet!

Dr. Joel Fuhrman, the writer of a variety of books including *Eat to Live, Super Immunity* and *The End of Diabetes*, treats his patients with arthritis with the equation of $H=N/C$ meaning Health is proportional to the Nutrient per Calorie density of your diet. Speaking about diet, Furhman says, "I have cared for hundreds of patients with rheumatoid arthritis, connective tissue disease, systemic lupus, fibromyalgia and other painful disorders. The vast majority of all these patients have been able to achieve complete remission or significant reduction in pain and need for medications. The majority of patients did not need to fast, but the most stubborn cases have found that periodic fasting was helpful for achieving long-term remission."

It never ceases to amaze me how the connection between our food and health is so prominent. Before becoming vegan, I never realized the connection except for weight loss. Now I know that I don't have to rely on the doctor for a simple cold; if I feel the symptoms soon enough I can combat that sucka with excellent nutrition, antibacterial & antiviral super herbs.

Type 2 Diabetes

Type 2 diabetes is sweeping over our country. This debilitating disease is completely preventable and curable with proper diet. According to the Physicians Committee for Responsible Medicine the first step to reversing diabetes is a vegan diet.

"Animal products contain fat, especially SATURATED fat, which is linked to heart disease, insulin resistance, and certain forms of cancer. These products also contain cholesterol, something never found in foods from plants. And, of course, animal products contain animal protein. It may surprise you to learn that diets high in animal protein can aggravate kidney problems and calcium losses. Animal products never provide fiber or healthful complex carbohydrate."

How to Survive in the Real World as a Vegan

OK, guys, now we are getting into the nitty-gritty of living the vegan life: facing the outside world! It's funny, you may have a buddy or acquaintance that will do destructive things like smoking, drugs and drinking. If you tell them that you are choosing to be a vegan all of a sudden that same person turns around and is all up in your face about it. This chapter will help you out in the real world from eating out to dealing with difficult people. At first, all of the questions that flew my way really bothered me, but I learned to accept these questions and even difficult people as an opportunity to educate.

Vegan blogger Sarah Eastin of healgrowblossom.com provides some insight on her experience in becoming vegan and resources she uses to thrive on a vegan lifestyle.

Most vegans I know have tons of energy, feel great almost every day of the year, feel good about their compassionate choice, eat amazing delicious foods, have minimized risk for diseases and lessen our environmental impact based on the foods we choose. I have found, however, that you really should do your research and learn how you can be vegan, healthy and thrive with this lifestyle. Don't go vegan without some thought.

Just a few of the resources that have helped along my journey include; attending healthy eating classes, reading all the books I can on healthy diet and lifestyle, research on the internet, networking with like-minded folks and exploring new restaurants and foods.

I take a multi vitamin and a B complex supplement. I am also conscious of my probiotic intake and try to drink Kombucha several times a week.

For recipes and meal ideas, I research recipes online and subscribe to several blogs, buy a few cookbooks here and there and check many out from the library. I also experiment with many different recipes and flavor combinations. One of my favorites is quesadillas, you can load them up with veggies, fruits, beans, nut butters, salsas, anything. I love 'em!

Going Out to Eat

Going out to eat can be a daunting task if you are eating a healthy diet or a specific diet like a vegan one. I used to be afraid that the waiter or chef would think I am being too picky when requesting a meal with numerous modifications. I then came to a realization that, "Hey! This is my body and I am in control of what goes in it!"

You are allowed to be as picky and ask as many questions as you want until you feel confident that you will get exactly what you want. Also, you are choosing to spend your hard-earned money at this particular eating establishment. Get what you want! We will review some terms that are generally safe on the menu for vegans and other terms to generally stay away from or how to modify them to become vegan.

Menu Terms to Avoid

As a whole avoid the following terms: creamy, cheese, battered and fried. Creamy normally implies it is made with dairy, cheese goes without saying, battered and fried you will need to ask the chef if the batter has egg or dairy in it. Typically what you can do is if you see the word creamy you can ask them to remove the cheese and replace the creamy sauce with a tomato-based or olive oil–based sauce instead. If the batter does contain egg or dairy you will need to forget all about the fried-ness because they normally are unable to adapt the batter to not include those ingredients. Here are some specific cuisines where you may run into trouble.

Mexican

Let's start with the rice. When ordering Mexican rice, ask them if it is made with vegetable broth or chicken broth. Many times Mexican restaurants cook their rice in chicken broth. When ordering any type of beans ask if they are cooked with pork or lard. Ask for them to cook any vegetable dish you order in oil instead of butter. Be sure to ask for NO cheese on any dish you order, sometimes they just assume that you want cheese even if it is not on the menu description. Stick to corn tortillas because many times the flour tortillas have dairy in them.

Italian

When enjoying Italian food, the main thing here is to make sure the dish does not have cheese in or on it. Many Italian restaurants have numerous vegan dishes or vegetarian dishes that can be made vegan so this is normally a good pick for vegans. When it comes to that scrumptious bread before the meal, ask if there is any dairy or egg in or on the bread. Also know that typically fresh hand-made pasta contain egg, just ask if you can have dry pasta instead.

Asian

As far as vegan-friendly cuisine Asian cuisines such as Thai, Chinese, Japanese, Vietnamese will normally always have something to enjoy. There are a couple of things to watch out for though. When ordering pad thai ask for the vegetable pad thai no egg and no fish sauce. Fish sauce is something you need to ask to remove each time from a veggie dish; besides that if you stick to the veggie menu options you are set.

Greek/Mediterranean

Greek restaurants normally have a variety of vegetarian dishes that can easily be made vegan if they are not already. In Mediterranean cooking, dairy in the form of cheese does sneak its way into veggie dishes so be sure to ask for no cheese. Some safe dishes are hummus, babaganoush and tabouleh. Dolmas are a good option too as long as they are not stuffed with beef so be careful when ordering these. Tzatiki and cucumber sauces normally have dairy in them so steer clear. Pita bread sometimes contains dairy so just ask.

Indian

Many Indian dishes are vegetarian but not all are vegan. Ghee is a clarified butter that is used in numerous dishes, so ask if the dish you want to order contains ghee. Paneer is an Indian cheese used in a variety of dishes. They also use cream in a variety of their vegetarian dishes. I recommend asking the waiter or chef which dishes have no dairy and stick to those. Some of their breads contain dairy so just double check before chowing down.

Quick Glance Out at Restaurants

Veg Friendly Preparation

Olive oil sauces

Sauté (double check it's cooked in oil not butter)

Tomato sauces

Roasted/baked

Danger Zone

Smothered – get the item un-smothered. Smothered typically

implies a gravy or cheese

Creamy – ask for a tomato or olive oil–based sauce instead

Cheesy – simply ask for the dish with no cheese, even pizza!

Crusted – just don't get it, they batter it up with egg and dairy

Fish sauce – only need to worry about in Asian restaurants

Vegan Restaurant Resources

https://www.vegguide.org/
http://www.vegdining.com/
www.happycow.net
www.yelp.com – type in vegan or vegetarian and your city

Smartphone Vegan Restaurant Locator Apps!

Animal-Free (FREE)

Happy Cow (FREE)

Roaming Hunger (FREE)

Vegan Xpress ($1.99)

Social Gatherings

Based on personal experience I have always enjoyed bringing something to a gathering for a couple of reasons. I enjoy cooking healthful, that way when someone asks how this was made I can give them a healthy recipe. I also enjoy contributing just for the joy of giving and being part of a gathering. Much of the same still holds true as a vegan.

Now that I am vegan I enjoy bringing a nice vegan side, entrée or dessert so that when people drool over it I can boast that it is vegan and give them a recipe. This opens their eyes that vegan food is delicious! It may also help people get off your back with vegan health questions. Next time you have a gathering I suggest bring killer chocolate chip cookies oozing with healthy coconut oil, almond meal, flax and chocolate chunks, of course. Or bring a fantastic slaw with maple tahini dressing.

If your party host insists that they are the ones to make your food I suggest giving them the link to some of your favorite recipes online or some recipes from this book! I suggest something healthy and well-rounded such as a dish with beans, grains, variety of veggies. And a little sweet treat so that you can be included at dessert time! Give them a simple recipe for raw chocolate truffles.

Traveling as a Vegan

From December 2015 – July 2016 I set off with my partner on a trip half way around the world. We began our journey in Colombia, continuing on to Ecuador, Peru, Indonesia, Thailand and Cambodia. We discovered that traveling as a vegan is actually the most affordable and healthful way to eat on the road. Although, it can have its challenges such as searching for food at a truck stop in Ecuador during an eight hour bus ride. My advice to traveling vegans is to shop at local markets, cook your own food when possible and give yourself a break. I will also share some of unique vegan finds in unsuspecting places.

Shop at Local Markets

Shopping at local markets is such a thrill! Shopping at local markets can teach a great deal about the local culture, customs and food. Unlike in the good ol' US of A, bargaining in

South America and South East Asia is expected. I enjoyed making a game out of it; some vendors are more willing to play than others. Haggling provides an opportunity to speak the local language and earn some respect from the locals. While some locations we skipped right on through, others we stayed for a couple of weeks or longer. Through repeat trips to the market, we learned who had the best deals and freshest produce. Imagine, you walk into a market in rural Peru, what is there for a vegan to buy?! Well, it turns out a lot! Much to my surprise, they had a huge variety of potatoes, vegetables and fruits. I was shocked to see they had the most beautiful, juicy fresh pomegranates.

Cook Your Own Food

Cooking while traveling enables you to save money and really connect with the food that you buy at the market. Many hostels have communal kitchens for guest use. Not only is the communal kitchen a place to cook, it is also a great place to meet others staying in the hostel. Preparing and cooking your meal is also much healthier. You control the amount of oil, type of oil, salt etc. that goes into your food. Additional accommodation options providing a kitchen include apartments, condos and houses. Thanks to the internet, you can filter for a kitchen. The accommodation websites we used most frequently are Booking.com and Airbnb.com.

Be Easy on Yourself

Give yourself a break! For the most part during our travels I was able to have great vegan snacks on hand like nuts and seeds, dried fruit, granola etc. However, seeing as this is real life, things do not always go according to plan. We found traveling by bus through South America to be the most affordable way to get around. One bus ride through Ecuador we ran out of healthy snacks. We were crazy hungry so at a truck stop we went inside to see what they had. The most veg friendly item they had was white rice mixed with what looked to be canned vegetables and shrimp. Well, you gotta eat right? So we grabbed a couple of those and ate around the shrimp. When traveling, you learn to adapt. In my mind, ordering a dish that has meat in it, and eating around the meat is better than having my blood sugar crash and getting the shakes. So, be easy on yourself.

Vegan Food Finds

During our travels we came across some incredible vegan food finds. During our stay in South America, we found the best value in food in Colombia. We experienced the largest, sweetest juiciest papaya I have ever had the pleasure of eating. They also have very large and flavorful pumpkin which we made three days' worth of meals from. Ecuador has beautiful fertile land allowing them to grow a vast variety of fruits and vegetables. They have decedent high quality chocolate made from the cacao plants of Ecuador. The market has a large variety of beans that made for interesting dishes.

In Peru we spent most of our time on the north coast where fresh mature coconuts are plentiful. We enjoyed drinking a coconut and eating the meat every day. One local vendor always had fresh ripe pomegranates. My favorite find in Peru has to be algarrobina syrup which is simply syrup made from the Black Carob tree. This native to Peru is high in iron, phosphorous, magnesium, potassium, vitamin A, vitamin B1, vitamin B2, vitamin D. It is also high in protein and natural sugar from the carob. It is a beautiful mild chocolate flavor. A dish we made almost every day in Peru was mashed up bananas, avocado, pomegranates and algarrobina syrup.

We began our stint in South East Asia in Indonesia followed by Thailand and Cambodia. South East Asia has a range of food, some familiar others not so much. We enjoyed our first taste of durian fruit. Durian goes by many names including "stinky fruit" and "king of fruits". It has an oddly beautiful flavor combination of sweet onions and cheesecake. All you have to do to find durian is to follow your nose. It has a pungent odor, which personally, I enjoy but many do not. The fruit is not allowed in public spaces such as hotels, train stations and airports. Durian is high in protein, B vitamins and fatty acids. Another fruit which happens to pair perfectly with durian is mangosteen fruit. It is a soft mild sweet fruit that is covered by a purple shell. The mildness of the fruit cuts through the richness of the durian making it a perfect pair. Another fruit we had the pleasure to enjoy is jackfruit. The fruit is contained in a large green balloon looking shell. The fruit itself are deep yellow bulbs. Jackfruit is an excellent source of vitamin C, B vitamins and fiber. South East Asia is a very friendly place for vegans, as most of their diet consists of rice and vegetables.

What Travel the Vegan Way Has to Say

My good friend and owner of Travel the Vegan Way, Sarah Vinz, she spent majority of her adult life traveling around the world experiencing different cultures and cuisines all as a vegan. If there are two things that excite Sarah Vinz, they would be being a vegan and traveling. She has been a vegetarian since she was a teenager, a vegan for the past ten years. She has lived, worked, and studied in nine countries (Germany, Guatemala, Kenya, Kosovo, the Netherlands, the Republic of Korea, Switzerland, Thailand, and Zambia), and travelled to over fifty more.

Sarsh created Travel the Vegan way to help other vegans see the world. If you would like to contact Sarah, she welcomes comments or questions at info@traveltheveganway.com. Visit her website at http://www.traveltheveganway.com!

Many people are a little intimidated by the thought of traveling as a vegan. In reality, it's nothing to be afraid of – it just may take a little bit of planning and research. The suggestions included in the "Going out to eat" section are a great starting point, and the list of vegan restaurant locator sites and apps will be an invaluable resource (probably even more on the road than while you are at home!). Here are a few tips and tricks that will help you make sure you get tasty, interesting, and nourishing vegan food while traveling.

Things to Pack

It's always a good idea to pack some nutrient-rich snacks, such as nuts, dried fruits, power bars, individual packs of oatmeal, and soup cups. These are especially important for those times when the range of options you have are limited – for instance, if you arrive at your hotel late in the evening and only have a vending machine to stave off hunger until morning. If you will be on a longer trip, you may also wish to bring a container of protein powder or some multi-vitamins, even if these products are not part of your regular daily routine. Your diet may be less in your control than it is at home, and it's important to ensure you are getting everything you need nutrition-wise.

Traveling by Air

If you are on an international flight, most airlines will provide special meals as long as the request is made in advance (usually 24 to 72 hours). Online ordering options sometimes exist, but I think it is safer to speak to an airline representative. When you call, explain that you are a vegan and do not eat any animal products. The agent should be able to guide you to the right meal choice (often "VGML") and read you a description of what the meal may or may not contain. Bear in mind that codes and terminology can vary between airlines. It's also a good idea to re-confirm your special meal request when you check in for your flight, and to stow some filling snacks in your carry-on in case there is an unexpected problem (such as a last-minute re-routing).

Most airports also now have a number of restaurants where vegan food is available. A quick google search of the city name plus "airport" and "vegan" will usually turn up a number of workable options. If you're pressed for time, head for the nearest burrito joint. Even Taco Bell offers vegan-friendly options!

Staying in Hotels

Many hotels offer a free breakfast these days. There will usually be at least a few vegan options that you can mix-and-match into a hearty breakfast, including fruit, bagels, bread, cereal, oatmeal, peanut butter, and juice. Hosts are usually quite willing to let you look at food labels, if this is a concern. My own tip is to try eating your cereal with juice instead of milk – it's actually pretty delicious! If you are staying more than a few days, you may wish to look for a hotel that offers some form of kitchen appliances, such as a mini-fridge, a coffee-maker (which in a pinch can be used to heat hot water for oatmeal or soup!), or a microwave. This will allow you to buy and prepare your own foods.

Tell Hosts and Travel Companions You Are Vegan

I think it's always a good idea to let anyone you might be spending time with on your trip know in advance that you are following a vegan lifestyle. If you are staying with people who are not familiar with what being a vegan entails, you might want to give them a short explanation of the foods you generally do and don't eat, so they know how to prepare for your visit. It can also be helpful to offer to do some of your own shopping upon arrival, or to cook up a vegan feast to share with everyone!

Work colleagues should be alerted in case they are planning

restaurant or working meals (often a quick email or telephone call to the person handling the logistical side of your visit will suffice). Conference planners should also be alerted if an event is catered. Vegan options can usually be arranged with advance notice.

Vegan Tourism

Lucky for us, the opportunities for vegans to take advantage of tours, cruises, and lodgings aimed specifically at plant-powered individuals are rapidly increasing in number. Taking advantage of these offerings means you are guaranteed to have a great array of vegan food, with little to no effort on your part! If you're looking for an organized tour, Veg Voyages offers tantalizing trips to India and Southeast Asia. If cruising is your thing, Holistic Holiday at Sea offers a week-long sailing to the Caribbean every March. And if you're looking for vegan or veg-friendly accommodation, a number of sites allow you to search by region, country, or city. A wonderful place to start for inspiration is *VegNews* magazine's online travel section.

Happy traveling!

Vegan Travel Resources

www.vegetarianguides.co.uk/products/ – To purchase the *Vegan Passport* and other Veg guides

www.happycow.net/ – Happy Cow's vegan travel forum

www.atasteofhealth.org/vegan-cruise – Holistic Holiday at Sea

www.vegvoyages.com

www.veggie-hotels.com

www.vegnews.com

Coming Out of the "Vegan" Closet

When I decided to become vegan I did not tell my family right away. Why, you ask? I decided to wait to tell them until I found my sweet spot. Remember that when I first became vegan I lost a lot of weight and did not feel my best. But once I found the right balance between nourishing my body with whole plant foods and fitness I felt strong and confident. I wanted them to look at me and be like damn...whatever she is doing, it is working, I want to do that! When I finally told them, it was in person over some kind of holiday or maybe it was a birthday.

Either way, I hadn't seen them for about 4 months or so, and once they were done telling me how great I looked I busted out that I was vegan. BAM! There was no way they could say ohhhh, you'll look sickly because clearly I wasn't, and they just got done doting over me after all. My family for the most part was and remains very supportive of my vegan choices.

They have certain concerns like how to have a healthy pregnancy while vegan. At the time I was not well equipped with oodles of information about vegan and pregnancy. Women are perfectly capable of having a healthy pregnancy, delivery and vegan children with proper nutrition and supplementation when necessary. Although they are supportive I still get grief that I am missing out on meat. I still do get annoyed but the subject drops pretty quick because they understand my core ethical reasons for being vegan.

Some things I have learned when telling people is that not to try and change them or persuade them that what you are doing is the "right" thing. I prefer to lead by example and they always seem to come around and ask for recipes and become genuinely interested. Some have even adopted a vegetarian or vegan life. It is important for you to stick to your core values of why you choose to live a vegan lifestyle. A lot of the time you find yourself in situations where you simply have to roll with the punches that people and life throw at you. You can't control others but you can control yourself and how you respond to situations. When you take the high road you are helping form a positive image of vegans.

Let's roll play again, shall we? Scenario, you are telling the person in your life who you are closest to, whether that be your mom, dad, friend, aunt or companion animals.

Special person: So this weekend for your birthday where do you want to go eat?

You: I was thinking of that new vegan restaurant in town, I hear their food is out of this world!

Special person: Vegan restaurant? You sure that's what you want? Not a nice steak dinner?

You: Well, I recently became vegan so a steak house probably wouldn't be the best option for me.

Special person: Mmmm-hmm... when did you become vegan and why did you decide to become vegan?

You: I started this lifestyle a couple months ago, and I decided that being vegan aligns best with my values. It no longer made sense for me to support a cruel industry when I strive to live a life with minimal harm as possible.

Special person: Interesting, but I care about you, and I always hear these horror stories about vegans dying from malnutrition. I just don't want you to die!

You: I appreciate your concern and can see where you got the misconception that vegans shrivel up and wilt away once eliminating animal products from their diet. Truth is, I feel stronger and more alive than ever before! I have now discovered so many new vegetables, grains and legumes and I never get bored. If you are interested we can do a cook-out for my birthday instead and I can share some of my new recipes.

Special person: Well, you do look great that's for sure! OK, I am willing to try some vegan recipes with you. Who knows, I may adopt the same.

OK, so the most important thing to remember is right here, right here on this card. You can print this off, take it with you to social gatherings, restaurants, or anywhere you may encounter a difficult situation.

Dealing with People

Since embarking on my vegan path I have come across three different types of people when you tell them you are vegan; the hard ass who just wants to be combative, the know-it-all who once you tell them you are a vegan they are suddenly a nutritionist, and the curious folks who really do just want to learn more. After we review how to deal with each type of person we will also dive into how to avoid feeling attacked and how to turn a tough situation into an educational experience instead.

The Hard Ass

So we all know these guys and gals, the hard asses. They are manly men because they eat meat. Or we didn't get to the top of the food chain for no reason. We all know this type of person. When you encounter a hard ass and they find out you are vegan there are a couple of ways to handle the situation.

Scenario 1: You are at a party with people you know and some you don't. This dude is waiting in line behind you for the food, he notices that you refused any meat. Ready, set, go!

Hard ass: Why aren't you having any steak, it looks amazing.

You: Oh, I am vegan and choose to not eat any meat.

Hard ass: So you don't eat ANY meat? What about chicken? Fish? Eggs? Cheese?! OMG I don't think I could survive without cheese.

You: Right, I do not eat any animals, land or sea, or anything that could come from an animal such as dairy and eggs. I instead focus on eating a huge variety of vegetables, nuts, grains, and fruits. I can't believe how amazing I feel since adopting a vegan diet.

In that particular situation it's best just to keep your cool and really elaborate on all of the new foods you get to eat and how great it has impacted your life.

Scenario 2: You are at a work birthday party that has ice cream and cake. A co-worker is trying to pressure you into eating some.

Hard ass: Have some cake and ice cream!

You: No, thank you.

Hard ass: Why not? You on a diet or something?

You: Actually no, I became vegan and no longer eat cake and ice cream made with dairy and eggs.

Hard ass: Well, there is no other way to make cake and ice cream besides with lots of butter, milk and eggs. You are going to starve! Sheesh, I can see you wilting away right now!

You: You are thinking "man, back off" but you keep your composure because you are awesome and you simply say well actually I have made quite a few different dessert recipes such as brownies and cookies by simply swapping the traditional butter with coconut oil, creating a flax egg instead of using real eggs and non-dairy milk instead of cow's milk. I can print you off some of my favorite recipes!

The Know-it-all

Gah...know-it-alls. Whether they are in our class, our jobs, or even in our circle of friends we have all come across a know-it-all at some point in our lives. These are the people who no matter what you say will always try and one up you to be right or to provide more information. With these types of people it is best to be prepared with the facts, from facts about factory farming to health. This is something that will come with time, but with the more research you do and the more you are active in your vegan community the easier this will become.

Scenario: You and the know-it-all are friends out at an eating establishment where they offer very minimal vegan options.

Know-it-all: Man...this burger looks sooooo good loaded with cheese and bacon. What are you thinking about getting?

You: Well, there aren't too many options for me, I could get the salad or maybe make up a dish with sides.

Know-it-all: What are you talking about? What about that chicken dish?

You: Well, since becoming vegan I have learned that sometimes you have to get creative when going out to eat.

Know-it-all: You are vegan?!?! Wow, that is so dangerous for your health! Vegans do not get nearly enough Iron in their diet to survive. They are also so tired and weak all of the time.

You: I understand where that misconception comes from that vegans do not get enough iron, with big agriculture telling us that we can only get iron from animals our whole lives. Really some of the top sources of iron come from dark green vegetables, soy and beans. Also, since becoming vegan I have experienced the complete opposite of tired. I feel full of life and energy all day long. I don't feel the need to reach for a cup of coffee in the afternoon or a sugary snack because I learned how to eat a variety of different plant foods to keep me energized all day.

In this situation you were able to handle yourself well with knowing where certain sources of vitamins and minerals come from. Like you are doing now, you are educating yourself and that really is the key to discussing veganism with people who are not and fed myths about being vegan.

When discussing veganism with people it is important to listen, empathize and use active listening techniques. If someone expresses how they feel they are afraid they wouldn't get enough protein you can say something along the lines of "I was also worried about not getting enough protein in my diet. I did some extensive research and found that protein is available in all plant foods, just some more than others including beans, lentils, cooked greens and soy."

If you are able to empathize with their concerns they will see that you are not perfect and shared the same concerns and will be interested in how you overcame them. Another technique to use with someone who is becoming defensive is to use "I" language..."I feel"..."I think"...etc. this way they are less likely to argue or tell you that what you feel is wrong. Remember that being comfortable talking about being vegan in social situations will get easier with time and practice.

What Do Vegans Eat?

You have made it to the most delicious part of the book, the recipes! Although this particular book is not intended to be a cookbook but more of a vegan starter book, I think it is appropriate to provide you with some delicious vegan recipes to get you off on the right foot. I compiled some of my favorite simple and oh-so-tasty recipes just for you!

One thing to keep in mind is that all of these recipes are omnivore tested and approved. Many of us whether we realize it or not, eat many vegan or almost vegan meals. I will provide tips on how to make some of your favorite meals vegan and how accessible and scrumptious a vegan diet really can be!

Breakfast aka Favorite Meal of the Day

Breakfast is my absolute favorite meal of the day, always has been and always will be. As a kid the only way my mom could get me out of bed was if I liked what was going to be served for breakfast that day. Today, before I go to bed I am looking forward to the next morning's meal because I know it will be amazing. Before being vegan my breakfast was cereal and almond milk or quick cooking oats. I was eating vegan breakfasts before and not even realizing it. Since becoming vegan my breakfast menu has expanded and gotten a whole lot more creative!

Favorite Meal of the Day Recipes

Kick Bootay Tofu Scramble

This is the type of recipe that gets made on special occasions or lazy weekend mornings. Not because it is labor intensive, it is actually quite simple, but I am more of a grains and smoothies type girl in the morning. For those who like a savory breakfast option or are removing eggs from their diet this is a great option.

Ingredients:

1 small yellow/sweet onion

2 cloves garlic diced

1 lb firm tofu pressed and crumbled

Handful of spinach chopped

2 roma tomatoes de-seeded and chopped

2 Tbs – ¼ cup nutritional yeast flakes

1 Tbs tamari or soy sauce

½ tsp turmeric

¼ tsp garlic powder

¼ tsp onion powder

1 tsp Dijon mustard

Salt and pepper to taste

Directions:

1. Press the water out of the tofu and crumble. Heat a large skillet over medium-high heat and add the oil and chopped onion and garlic. Sauté until translucent.

2. Add in your tofu and all spices except the salt and pepper and sauté for about 5-7 minutes. Taste test then salt and pepper to taste. At the end of the cooking add in your tomatoes and spinach until just wilted.

3. Serve with some tempeh bacon, fruit or put in a wrap for a killer burrito.

Sweet N' Smoky Tempeh Bacon

I am in love with tempeh bacon. Before I was vegan I always preferred bacon to sausage. I have to say that this tempeh bacon rocks the pants off of traditional bacon. I just love the flavor combination; it makes my mouth water just thinking about it. I love to serve this alongside some tofu scramble or in a burrito, on top of salads, in sandwiches or straight off the skillet. I hope you enjoy this as much as I do!

Ingredients:

1 8 oz package tempeh

1 Tbs Grade B maple syrup

1 Tbs olive oil

Smidgen cayenne pepper

1 tsp liquid smoke

1 tsp tamari or soy sauce

Couple teaspoons olive oil for pan sauté

Directions:

1. Very thinly slice the tempeh.

2. Combine all of the ingredients in a large baggie.

3. Throw the tempeh in the bag with the liquid mixture and gently mix it all up making sure each slice gets a nice coating of the sauce.

4. Seal the bag, stick it in the fridge for at least 1 hour preferably overnight.

5. When you are ready to make the tempeh, heat a skillet over medium heat with the olive oil.

6. Sauté the marinated tempeh for 1 minute or so on each side until the sides are all nice and caramelized.

7. Serve with tofu scramble, on sandwiches, wraps, or all by itself, and enjoy!

Basic Vegan Pancakes

Pancakes are something I enjoy making on occasion, maybe serve your honey something special in bed one day. I provided the basic vegan pancake base. But think of pancakes as a canvas; add any kinds of spices, fruits, nuts and seeds to these guys. Also get creative with the toppings. I provided a few options but another great one is mashed banana used as a sauce. Enjoy!

Ingredients:

1 cup flour of choice – I really enjoy unbleached all-purpose flour, whole wheat pastry flour and spelt flour

1 Tbs cane sugar

2 tsp baking powder

1 tsp salt

1 cup non-dairy milk; I prefer soy or almond

2 Tbs melted coconut oil or vegetable oil

Add-Ins which I totally recommend

1 tsp ground ginger

1 tsp cinnamon

½ tsp nutmeg

1 tsp vanilla extract

1 tsp almond extract

Blueberries and walnuts

Pumpkin puree and dark chocolate chips

Directions:

1. Heat a medium skillet over medium heat.

2. Combine all of your dry ingredients and pour in your non-dairy milk and oil. Combine but don't overmix.

3. Fold in any optional add-ins.

4. Spray the pan with some non-stick cooking spray and pour on one ice cream scoop worth of batter on pan.

5. When you see bubbles start to pop at the top of the pancake or if the edges start to stiffen, carefully flip over. Cook for about 3 more minutes on the other side.

6. I treat the first pancake as a test to see if I need to cook the pancake a bit more or less.

7. Pour over some warmed maple syrup with some Earth Balance butter. Or top with some thinned nut butter and banana slices. It's your creation, go crazy!

Zucchini Bread Oatmeal

So this is a new obsession of mine. Before becoming vegan my oats consisted of quick cooking oats, in the microwave with water and counting calories like a mad woman. Now, I load my oats up with a variety of different toppings and fruits. If you are not a huge fan of zucchini you can shred carrots or sweet potatoes in here as well to make a carrot cake oatmeal or sweet potato oatmeal. To. Die. For.

Ingredients:

½ cup whole rolled oats

1 cup non-dairy milk; I love coconut milk or vanilla soy milk for a creamy recipe

1 small or ½ large zucchini shredded

1 tsp coconut oil

1 banana mashed

1 tsp grade b maple syrup

½ tsp cinnamon

¼ tsp nutmeg

¼ tsp ground ginger

1 tsp pure vanilla extract

Toppings

1 Tbs walnuts

1 Tbs raisins

Sprinkle of cinnamon

Drizzle of maple syrup

Directions:

1. Heat a pot over medium-low heat.

2. Shred your zucchini while pot is heating up.

3. Melt the coconut oil and add your shredded zucchini, sauté for a couple of minutes until fragrant.

4. Now add in your rolled oats and non-dairy milk and cook for about 10 minutes. You'll need to keep an eye on things in case the oats boil over or the milk starts to stick to the bottom, so stir once in a while.

5. Once you see things start to thicken up add in your mashed banana, spices and maple syrup.

6. When the oats are to your liking of thickness turn off the heat and stir in your vanilla extract.

7. Pour into a bowl and put the toppings on; enjoy your nice comforting bowl of oats!

Favorite Green Smoothie

It took me a while to get into green smoothies but I needed a quick way to ensure that I got my daily dose of greens in for the day. I suggest starting off with a couple cups of spinach. You can bump up the amount of greens you put in a smoothie.

WARNING! There will come a point where you can taste that there is too much greens in there. With practice and experience you will find that sweet spot with green smoothies. For the most part, you will not be able to taste the greens mixed in with everything else. Trust me on this one, guys.

Ingredients:

1 cup non-dairy milk; I like almond milk for this recipe

1 Tbs almond butter or other favorite nut butter

1 Tbs chia seeds

2 giant handfuls of baby spinach or 3 large kale leaves torn small

1 frozen banana

Directions:

1. Pour in your almond milk followed by the almond butter, chia seeds, greens and topped with the frozen banana.

2. Blend. Pour. Foodgasm.

Peaches N' Cream Smoothie

Mmmmm, who doesn't love peaches with cream? If you are one of those people who don't, you can transform this into a strawberries and cream smoothie instead. Anyways, I absolutely love seasonal peaches. The peaches here in Colorado are outstanding, so take advantage of those summer peaches. If they are out of season I recommend using frozen peaches instead.

Ingredients:

1 cup coconut milk

1 large ripe juicy peach or ½ cup frozen peaches

1 frozen banana

1-2 dates

2 Tbs cashews

Directions:

Add in the coconut milk, cashews, dates, and fruit. Blend it up until smooth and enjoy the bliss!

Go-To Overnight Oats

When I was working early mornings I would make these the night before in some Tupperware. They are nutritionally packed and taste so creamy, they are something definitely worth waking up for in the morning.

Ingredients:

½ cup rolled oats

1 cup non-dairy milk of choice

1 Tbs chia seeds

1 tsp cinnamon

1 tsp vanilla extract

Topping Ideas

1. 1 Tbs favorite nut butter

2. Coconut flakes

3. Fruit such as blueberries

4. Chopped nuts and dried cherries

Directions:

1. Combine all of the ingredients together in a bowl and cover in the fridge overnight. In the morning you will wake up to a beautiful bowl of creamy dreamy oats. Devour!

Breakfast Ice Cream

Ice cream for breakfast...say what?! That's right! This is a great breakfast option for kids and picky eaters. It is quite a fun twist on breakfast to wake up to the creamy guilt-free ice cream. Go wild with any mix-ins and toppings. Pretend it's a healthy frozen yogurt shop!

Ingredients:

2 frozen bananas

About ¼ cup non-dairy milk but start small so the mixture isn't too liquidy.

Mix-ins:

Nut butter

Nut butter + jam (almond butter + raspberry jam)

Fruits

Cocoa powder

½ avocado

Directions:

1. Chop up the frozen bananas and add to a food processor and begin to pulse.
2. Add in the non-dairy milk as needed to help the bananas process. When things start to meld together add in your mixes.
3. Once all combined, pour into a bowl and eat like that or top with your favorite vegan granola.

Layered Cherry Banana Soft Serve and Chocolate Overnight Oats

Oh man, we are combining my all-time favorite flavors of cherries and chocolate. On top of that they are layered between each other making for the most indulgent yet healthy parfait. I absolutely love this breakfast, or have it as an afternoon snack. Heck, have it any time of day!

Ingredients:

Oats

½ cup rolled oats

1 cup non-dairy milk of choice

1 Tbs cocoa or cacao powder

1 Tbs chia seeds

1 tsp cinnamon

1 tsp vanilla extract

Banana Soft-Serve

1 frozen banana

½ cup slightly thawed frozen cherries or fresh

About ¼ cup non-dairy milk but start small so the mixture isn't too liquidy.

Directions:

1. Combine all of the overnight oat ingredients together in a bowl and cover overnight in the fridge.
2. In the morning combine all of the soft-serve ingredients together in a food processor. In a nice tall glass alternate between layering your overnight oats and soft-serve. Now literally dig in!

Chia Seed Pudding

Chia seeds! Woot! Woot! Remember chia pets? Those come from these seeds, how cool is that?! Chia seeds are extremely versatile and I love them in pudding. You can serve this pudding as breakfast or a nice healthy treat after dinner or even a great post-workout snack. If you don't dig the texture of the chia seed pudding, try blending them or using a spice grinder to make the texture more silky.

Ingredients:

¼ cup chia seeds

1 cup non-dairy milk

1 banana thinly sliced

1 tsp vanilla extract

1-2 tsp sweetener such as agave or pure maple syrup

Directions:

1. Whisk the seeds and milk together or else the chia seeds can clump up together and that doesn't look, taste or feel appealing.
2. Add in the vanilla extract, sweetener and banana.
3. Let everything dance in the fridge for at least 15 minutes. However I suggest letting sit for a few hours or even overnight so it can be ready in the morning for ya!

Lunch aka Middle of the Day Eating

For many Americans including myself, lunch is all about quick, convenient and nutritious eating. I like to utilize dinner leftovers from the night before in my lunch either by topping a salad with them, tossing it in a wrap or just eating straight leftovers.

Thankfully for these mid-day meals my leftover lunches turn from lame to outta' this world good. The Classic Vegan Ruben, Over-Stuffed Veggie Wrap and Rainbow Salad, lunch time is anything but boring.

Middle of the Day Eating Recipes

Classic Vegan Reuben

OK, to be honest, I used to despise Reuben sandwiches. All of the sourness in between two slices of bread was not happening for me. That all changed when I made my own vegan version. Gosh, at first bite this blew my taste buds away! The slightly sweet flavor of the tempeh combined with the warmed sauerkraut and creamy avocado feels like heaven in your mouth. I hope you like it as much as I do!

Ingredients:

Tempeh: use the Sweet N' Smoky Tempeh Bacon recipe

Sandwich

2 slices crusty bread such as sourdough, multi-grain loaf, or Italian bread, sliced

1 ripe avocado

1 small tomato thinly sliced

¾ cup sauerkraut

Vegan mayo such as Veganaise

Thousand Island Dressing

1 Tbs Vegenaise

1 tsp agave syrup

Dash of paprika

Dash of cayenne pepper or ¼ tsp horseradish

Directions:

1. Prepare all of your veggies and toast your bread. Also be warming up a skillet over medium heat.

2. Add a little bit of oil in the pan and cook the tempeh until both sides are nice and warmed. Remove the tempeh from the pan and add the sauerkraut to warm it through a bit.

3. On one slice of toasted bread spread the mayo over and the other slice spread your thousand island dressing.

4. Now add the tempeh, tomato, avocado slices and sauerkraut. This makes a monster of a sandwich...but that's how I like them, big and messy. Share with a friend, or not. It's up to you.

Over-Stuffed Veggie Wrap

This is a typical lunch for me, something simple that I can just dig around in my fridge, find the ingredients and throw them into a wrap. Be sure to get a variety of veggies so you can get all those vital nutrients!

Ingredients:

1 sprouted grain wrap½ avocado sliced

1 tsp whole grain mustard

1 small tomato

2 Tbs hummus

Handful of sprouts

Some spinach torn up small

Some shredded carrots

Directions:

1. Warm the tortilla in a skillet for a few minutes so it can bend easily.

2. Spread on the hummus, mustard and avocado slices

3. Now add the rest of the veggies.

4. Fold the two smaller sides of the wrap and then roll it all together.

Rainbow Salad

When I make a salad I don't stop at a little bit of greens and a dressing. Oh no! When you have a salad of mine you have a fest in a bowl. This salad is not only a treat to your mouth but it is beautiful with the contrast of colors from the purple cabbage to the red bell peppers.

Ingredients:

1 cup de-stemmed kale torn into small pieces

1 cup shredded or chopped red cabbage

1 cup chopped rainbow chard

½ red bell pepper chopped

1 apple thinly sliced

½ cup sauerkraut

1 Tbs chopped pecans

1 Tbs chopped walnuts

Dressing:

¼ cup extra virgin olive oil

2 Tbs balsamic vinegar

1 tsp whole grain mustard

1 tsp orange zest

Salt and pepper to taste

Directions:

1. Combine all of the salad ingredients.

2. Evenly distribute dressing over the salad, dig in and enjoy a real vegan salad, not a measly iceberg and tomato salad.

Creamy Mushroom Melt

This for me is comfort food in between bread. I love how aromatic the mushrooms and onions smell and then combined with the creamy melty Daiya cheese this is a sandwich you will crave time and time again.

Ingredients:

2 cups thinly sliced mushrooms

½ cup thinly sliced shallots

½ Tbs olive oil

¼ cup vegetable stock

Fresh parsley

Salt and pepper

Daiya mozzarella shreds

Crusty bread such as sourdough or nice crusty whole-grain bread

Directions:

1. In a large skillet over medium-high heat, add the olive oil, shallots and mushrooms. Sauté for about 5 minutes until browned. Add in the vegetable stock and simmer until reduced. Take off heat and add your salt, pepper and parsley.

2. Get your bread and pile on the mushroom mixture and top with the Daiya cheese shreds. Put the sandwich in a Panini press. If you don't have a Panini press you can simply put the sandwich in a hot pan and press down with a heavy book, flip and repeat.

Enjoy the ooey gooey sandwich!

Black Bean Sweet Potato Wrap

Ah yes, more simple delicious lunch wraps. The combo of sweet potato and black beans is just like peanut butter and chocolate. If you don't want to wait for the potato to bake you can chop and boil for about 15-20 minutes. I do, however, love how the sweet potato gets all silky, sweet and sticky with its own juices. Oh man, anyways, just throw these ingredients all together in a wrap and gobble it up.

Ingredients:

1/3 cup black beans

1 sweet potato baked

1 sprouted whole grain wrap

½ avocado sliced

Spinach sliced thin

1 Tbs cilantro finely chopped

Salsa

Directions:

1. This is super easy to throw together, especially if the potato is pre-baked. Simply throw in a 450 degree oven for about 45 minutes or until you can easily pierce with a fork.
2. Warm up your tortilla real quick on the stove top or the microwave.
3. Add some sweet potato, the avocado, cilantro, black beans, spinach and top with salsa.
4. Fold in the sides of the tortilla and wrap it up and stick it in your mouth. Chew. Smile. Repeat!

Marinated Kale Salad

So many people get turned off by kale because of its potential bitter taste. Well you know what, I don't really like the taste of straight up raw kale myself. I have to massage it with a beautiful dressing and all of a sudden it is outstanding! Couple of tips for kale is to not eat the stem, tear into small pieces and massage with a dressing and let sit for 10-30 minutes.

Ingredients:

1 bunch kale, de-stemmed

2 Tbs olive oil

3 Tbs lemon juice

2 Tbs tamari

2 Tbs nutritional yeast

2 Tbs hemp seeds

Directions:

1. De-stem and tear kale into small pieces.

2. Wisk together the dressing (remaining ingredients) and pour over kale.

3. Massage kale leaves with the dressing with your hands; this is fun!

4. Let the salad sit for at least ten minutes in the fridge. Now add any additional toppings such as fruits and seeds, even grains such as brown rice and quinoa.

Colorful Buddha Bowl

All a "Buddha bowl" is, is a nice grain such as quinoa or brown rice with a light dressing and a bountiful amount of fresh raw veggies. The key to this Buddha bowl is chopping the veggies up nice and small. I always feel so energized and Zen after eating one of these. Nourish your body and soul with this lunch.

Ingredients:

Salad

1 cup quinoa

1 carrot diced

½ red bell pepper diced

1 green onion thinly sliced

½ cup chickpeas

½ cup cherry tomatoes halved

½ avocado chopped

Dressing

1 lemon juiced

2 Tbs tamari

Sea salt to taste

Couple dashes of cayenne pepper

Directions:

1. To get 1 cup of cooked quinoa combine ½ cup dry quinoa with 1 cup of water, bring to a boil, reduce heat to simmer and cover for 20 minutes.

2. While the quinoa is cooking chop all of your vegetables and whisk together your dressing.

3. Toss the quinoa and vegetables together and add dressing.

4. Feel the Zen!

Dinner aka Memory Making Food

My next favorite meal has to be dinner. I love the feeling of taking time to unwind in the evening after a long day to get creative in the kitchen. I love the smell of a casserole baking, soup simmering on the stovetop or a beautiful veggie sauté and brown rice. If you have a significant other or family, get them in the kitchen with you. This is where wonderful memories are made. If you are solo take this time to reflect on the day and enjoy being with the awesomeness that is you.

Memory Making Food Recipes

Mighty Mushroom Pizza

So many people think that their lives might as well just be over without pizza. Hence, they use that as a crutch to not become vegan. Well, well, people, let me tell you, vegan pizza rocks! As a kid I would actually do this weird thing where I would scrape all the topping off the pizza including the cheese and just eat the dough with pizza sauce on it. As an adult you can see I still dig pizza cheeseless! I will admit, though, a bit of Daiya cheese is a nice touch! You can find the Field Roast sausage either in the refrigerated section with the tofu or in the freezer section with the meatless options.

Ingredients:

1 pizza crust

½ - 1 cup pizza sauce of choice; I really like Organicville brand

1 cup sliced mushrooms

½ cup thinly sliced red bell pepper

2 Italian Field Roast sausages thinly sliced

Daiya cheese (optional)

Directions:

1. Pre-heat the oven to what the pizza crust package says.

2. Prepare the veggies and Field Roast.

3. Spread a thin layer of sauce over the pizza crust, top with the remaining ingredients.

4. I really enjoy a pizza without cheese, even vegan cheese, but if you prefer, spread on some mozzarella or cheddar Daiya cheese.

5. Bake pizza according to directions and sprinkle on some nutritional yeast at the end.

Spring Lemony Leek Quinoa

Before becoming vegan I had never even heard of leeks - tragic, right?! When spring rolls around I really start to crave light fun vibrant dishes like this one! I hope that you enjoy the beautiful lemony dressing as much as I do.

Ingredients:

1 cup quinoa rinsed and drained

1 leek washed and thinly sliced

½ cup frozen peas

½ cup strawberries thinly sliced

Dressing

2 lemons juiced

¼ cup extra virgin olive oil

Salt and pepper to taste

Directions:

1. Bring a pot to medium heat and add the sliced leeks and sauté for about 3-5 minutes.

2. Add the quinoa and 2 cups of water and bring to a boil; once a boil is reached cover and simmer for 20 minutes.

3. 15 minutes into the quinoa cooking add the frozen peas and strawberries.

4. Add the dressing and mix while warm.

Over-Stuffed Sweet Tater

I am obsessed with sweet potatoes. I am telling you, OBSESSED!

Growing up, the only time I would have sweet potatoes at my house was during the holidays smothered with butter, brown sugar and mushrooms. Now I enjoy using sweet taters as a vessel for kick-ass toppings like this savory broccoli and mushroom mixture.

Ingredients:

1 medium sweet potato

½ cup mushrooms chopped

1 cup broccoli pieces chopped

Dressing

2 Tbs vegenaise

1 Tbs sweet potato

Dash of chipotle powder

1 tsp pure maple syrup

Directions:

1. Pre-heat oven to 450 degrees. Pierce potato with a knife a few times, wrap with foil and place in oven about 45 minutes, flipping after 30 minutes.

2. While the potato is cooking chop up your broccoli and mushrooms. Heat a skillet over medium heat and add the broccoli, sauté for about 8 minutes. Add some water and

do a quick broccoli steam. Add in your mushrooms at the end of the broccoli cooking.

3. When the potato is ready open and scoop out a tablespoon of tater meat and combine with the dressing ingredients.

4. Now compile that sucka! Split the tater in half, add your broccoli mushroom mix on top, then spread the sauce over the top of it all. DEVOUR!

Mac N' Cheeze Baby

I used to not really be into macaroni and cheese. I thought it was super lame, kinda boring and didn't really taste like cheese. You know what I'm talking about, the boxed stuff with the dinosaur on the package. Anyways, after learning how to make creamy vegan cheese with cashews as the base my attitude towards this classic has drastically changed. Try it, you won't even miss the dairy!

Ingredients:

1 package pasta of choice

Cheeze Sauce

1 cup raw cashews soaked overnight

¼ cup unsweetened non-dairy milk

½ - ¾ cup nutritional yeast

½ tsp garlic powder

¼ tsp onion powder

2 tsp tamari

Directions:

1. Cook pasta according to package directions; I aim for al dente.

2. Drain and rinse the cashews. While the pasta is cooking start to prepare the sauce in a blender. Adjust seasonings to taste.

3. Pour sauce into a pot and warm through.

4. Drain pasta and pour sauce on pasta. Serve and sprinkle on some paprika for some nice flavor and color contrast. We eat with our eyes first!

Italian Quinoa Pasta with Broccolini

I love going to the store and finding something I've never seen before. I remember seeing broccolini on the Food Network and thought they were just adorable and had to find them! Broccolini really just look like skinny baby broccoli. They only take a couple of minutes to cook and look delicate and impressive to guests.

Ingredients:

1 package quinoa pasta

½ Tbs extra virgin olive oil

1 bunch broccolini or broccoli chopped small

1 small sweet onion chopped

2 cloves garlic diced

1 pint cherry or grape tomatoes

¼ cup sun-dried tomatoes chopped

¼ cup fresh basil torn

Directions:

1. Prepare quinoa pasta according to directions; be sure to not overcook.

2. Prepare all of your veggies, heat a skillet over medium heat.

3. Add the oil, onions and garlic and sauté for about 5 minutes or until translucent. Next add in your broccolini or broccoli and cook until fork tender.

4. Add in your cherry tomatoes and crush them a bit in the pan and add the sun-dried tomatoes. At the very end, stir in the torn basil.

5. Drain your pasta and add to the skillet with all of the veggies and combine.

6. Serve immediately and gobble up!

Colorful Warming Stew

I love stews. There, I said it. With this recipe you can really throw in any veggies you may have on hand. This stew is brimming with beautiful vibrant colors that our bodies crave so badly during the winter months. If you are under the weather this is also a fabulous recipe to help your body heal. With all of the different colors in one bowl you know it is jam-packed with vitamins and antioxidants to kick that illness in the butt!

Ingredients

2 cups vegetable broth

2 Tbs extra virgin olive oil

1 15 oz can diced tomatoes

2 carrots chopped

1 sweet onion chopped

1 red bell pepper chopped

2 cloves garlic chopped

1 zucchini chopped

1 cup grain of choice such as farro rinsed

1 cup edamame de-shelled

1 tsp coriander

1 tsp cinnamon

½ tsp garlic powder

Salt and pepper to taste

2 Tbs lemon juice

3 Tbs chopped fresh parsley

Directions:

1. Get a big ol' soup pot and bring to medium heat.

2. Chop all of those scrumptious veggies and rinse your grains.

3. Add the olive oil, onions, and garlic and sauté for about 5 minutes until fragrant. Now add the remaining veggies except the edamame and sauté for about 7 minutes.

4. Add the spices, vegetable broth, tomatoes and rinsed grains and bring to a boil. Once brought to a boil reduce heat to a simmer and cover for about 20 minutes. Do keep an eye on it, though, and add water to help thin it out if needed.

5. After 20 minutes stir in the edamame, lemon juice, chopped parsley and salt and pepper to taste.

6. Pour into bowls and serve with toasted crusty bread with vegenaise spread all over.

Black Bean Sweet Potato Burgers

I do love making burgers, especially during the warm summer months with friends and family. These sweet potato black bean burgers are full of beautiful flavors, vitamins and fiber to rock your world! Serve these with some purple cabbage slaw and you've got yourself a backyard BBQ winner!

Ingredients:

1 sweet potato

1 15 oz can black beans, rinsed and drained

½ cup oat flour or oat bran

1 flax egg (1 Tbs ground flax + 3 Tbs water)

½ tsp cinnamon

½ tsp cumin

¼ tsp coriander

Salt and pepper

Whole grain or sprouted grain burger buns

Toppings

Sliced tomatoes

Greens

Avocado

Condiments of choice such as BBQ sauce, hummus, vegenaise,

whole grain mustard, etc.

Directions:

1. Bake sweet potato in 450 degree oven 40-45 minutes.

2. Rinse and drain the beans and put into a bowl, mash up a bit with a potato masher or a fork, still leaving some beans whole.

3. Prepare the flax egg and set aside.

4. Scoop the meat from the sweet potato and add to the beans. Also add the oat flour, spices and flax egg. Combine well.

5. Heat a skillet over medium heat. While that is heating, form the mixture into 4-6 patties, depending on the size.

6. Spray the skillet with non-stick spray and put the patties on for about 4-6 minutes each side.

7. Toast the buns and get toppings ready.

8. Compile the burger: bottom bun with hummus spread on it topped with the burger patty, greens, sliced tomatoes, sliced avocado and top bun spread with BBQ sauce.

Dessert

I'm gonna be honest with you, if I reach for dessert it is typically a few squares of dark chocolate or coconut ice cream from the freezer. I do, however, have a few tricks up my sleeve when it comes to dessert. I really enjoy packing in some nutrition into my desserts as well, so that you don't have to feel guilty, right?

Dessert Recipes

Cinnamon Apples with Almond Butter Sauce

You've had your amazing vegan dinner but have a little craving for something sweet and healthy. These quick cinnamon apples are a perfect dessert at the end of a long day. The creamy coconut oil with the warming spices brings these apples to life! Top with a bit of almond butter and I am as happy as a bug in a rug.

Ingredients:

1 apple of choice; I love honeycrisp!

1/2 Tbs coconut oil

½ tsp cinnamon

¼ tsp ground ginger

Pinch sea salt

Pinch nutmeg

1 Tbs almond butter

Directions:

1. Chop the apple and place in a microwave safe bowl.

2. Top the apple with coconut oil and spices.

3. Microwave for 1-2 minutes stirring halfway through cook time.

4. Top with almond butter and enjoy this healthy dessert.

Secret Ingredient Chocolate Pudding

This was one of the first vegan desserts that I made. I never knew that you could use an avocado as the creamy base for pudding. If everyone knew this I don't think puddings would ever be made the same again. The coconut flavor is quite pronounced in this pudding which I love but if you need to you can cut back on the oil.

Ingredients:

1 avocado

2 Tbs almond butter

¼ cup cacao powder

1 Tbs coconut oil

2 Tbs agave syrup

Couple splashes of non-dairy milk to help combine.

Directions:

1. Combine all of the ingredients together in a food processor; add milk as needed to help blend.

2. Chill mixture for at least an hour before serving.

Pumpkin Pie Mousse

I made this dessert for Thanksgiving one year and it rocked my world! I even made enough that I could enjoy it for breakfast the next day. Be sure to purchase pumpkin pie puree, NOT pumpkin pie mix in the can. This pie goes awesome with some store bought vegan whipped cream or you can even make your own - it really is super easy!

Pie Ingredients:

1 15 oz canned pure pumpkin

1 package water-packed silken soft tofu, pressed

2 Tbs pure maple syrup

1 tsp pumpkin pie spice

1 tsp vanilla extract

Whipped Cream Ingredients:

1 can full fat coconut milk

1 tsp pure vanilla extract

1-2 tsp maple syrup or agave nectar

Directions:

1. Press the tofu so water comes out.

2. Break up the tofu and add to either a blender or food processor. Add in the pumpkin puree, maple syrup and pumpkin pie spice. Blend. Taste test and adjust sweetness and spice as desired.

3. Chill in fridge for at least 1 hour before serving. Pour into pretty glasses and top with vegan whipped cream.

4. For the coconut whipped cream, put the can of coconut milk in fridge over-night. In the morning flip the can over and pour the milk into a bowl and scoop out the coconut cream into a cold bowl. Whip the coconut cream until nice and fluffy, add in the vanilla extract and sweetener.

Simply Raw Chocolate

Can you tell I like simple yet delectable desserts yet? Ever thought it would be too hard to make your own chocolate? I thought so, until I realized how combining just a few ingredients and a freezer can change all of that!

Ingredients:

2 Tbs coconut oil, softened

2 Tbs cacao powder

½ tsp agave syrup

Directions:

1. Combine all ingredients by hand until silky smooth.

2. Pour onto a plate lined with parchment paper, pour mixture and spread.

3. Place in freezer for at least 20 minutes until firm enough to break into pieces.

Sexy Decadent Walnut Fudge

At first bite I am pretty sure I went into a blissful state of euphoria. If you want to impress your non-veg friends and family with a dessert, this will certainly win them over. In my opinion this fudge tastes way better than its dairy counterpart. I don't even have the words to truly describe the beauty that is this dessert, you will just have to make it. Now. Go make it now.

Ingredients:

½ cup coconut oil

¼ cup almond butter or nut butter of choice

½ cup cacao powder

½ cup pure maple syrup or agave syrup

1 Tbs pure vanilla extract

Pinch of fine sea salt

½ cup walnuts chopped

Directions:

1. Combine the coconut oil and nut butter with beaters or by hand.

2. Add in the cacao powder and beat that in there too.

3. Add the maple syrup, vanilla extract and sea salt and combine.

4. Now stir in the chopped walnuts, reserving some to put on top of the fudge.

5. Line a loaf pan with parchment paper and pour chocolate mixture into pan. Top with reserved walnuts. Stick in freezer for at least 1 hour. Once firm enough cut into squares.

Sauces, Condiments and Dressings

This was an interesting stage in my healthy eating journey, reading the back of the labels on ketchup, marinades, etc. There were all sorts of ingredients that I could not pronounce and high fructose corn syrup. Gross! So I switched to all organic brands or sauces and condiments, but over time this gets to become a bit pricey. So I decided to start making my own. At first I found this intimidating, but once you find your favorite flavor combinations they are quick to whip up, healthy for you and healthy for your wallet.

Sauces, Condiments and Dressings Recipes

Creamy Avocado Sauce

I was a little leery of the sound of this sauce at first but once all of the ingredients are melded together it is a beautiful creamy flavorful sauce. I love it on top of pasta or spaghetti squash.

Ingredients:

1 large ripe avocado

1 large lemon juiced

2 cloves garlic

¼ cup fresh basil

Salt and pepper to taste

Directions:

1. Chop the garlic up a bit.

2. Place all of the ingredients into a food processor and blend until well incorporated.

3. Pour on top of fresh hot pasta or use as a spread on wraps and sandwiches!

Vegan Ranch Dressing

Traditional ranch dressing is quite low on my list of favorite dressings. However, making your own vegan version will rock the pants off of any ranch dressings of the past.

Ingredients:

½ cup raw cashews soaked overnight

3 Tbs lemon juice

1/8 tsp garlic powder

1/8 tsp onion powder

¼ cup fresh parsley

¼ cup green onions

1 Tbs tahini

½ tsp Dijon mustard

½ cup water

1 tsp agave syrup

½ tsp salt

1/8 tsp black pepper

Directions:

1. Soak cashews in water overnight and drain and rinse in the morning.

2. Add the ingredients into a blender, blend until smooth.

3. Enjoy on any salad or wrap!

Vegan "Cheeze"

People can no longer use the excuse of they love cheese too much to become vegan because you can make your very own vegan cheese without all the nastiness of dairy. Soaked cashews make for an excellent base for the creamy cheesy sauce.

Ingredients:

1 cup raw cashews soaked overnight

½ cup nutritional yeast

1 tsp Dijon mustard

¼ tsp onion powder

¼ tsp garlic powder

1/8 tsp chili powder

½ tsp salt

¼ tsp black pepper

Directions:

1. Drain and rinse the cashews.

2. Add all ingredients into a blender and whirl around until nice and smooth.

Cashew Cream

This is the base recipe for cashew cream. You can take this basic recipe and make into a savory sauce or a sweet dessert cream. Play around with some different ingredients to find what you like the best. I really love this base mixed with fresh basil, parsley and tomatoes!

Ingredients:

1 cup cashews soaked overnight

2 Tbs lemon juice

¼ tsp salt

1 tsp sweetener such as agave nectar or maple syrup

Directions:

1. Drain and rinse the cashews.

2. Add all ingredients into a blender and whirl around until nice and smooth.

Peanut Ginger Sauce

I love getting the peanut dipping sauce for my spring rolls at Thai restaurants. Now you can make a beautiful peanut ginger sauce like you would find at your favorite Asian restaurant. Another nice thing is that you control the quality of ingredients so it's not over packed with sodium leaving you bloated at the end of the meal. Ewwwww.

Ingredients:

½ cup water

½ cup smooth unsalted peanut butter

1 Tbs rice wine vinegar

2 tsp tamari

2 tsp agave syrup

2 tsp fresh ginger grated

2 cloves garlic minced

Directions:

1. Whisk together all of the ingredients in a bowl and serve as a sauce for noodles, rice and veggies!

2. If you want things a bit spicier add a teaspoon of chili sauce.

Importance of Seasonal Eating

There is almost nothing I love better than waking up to a nice spring or summer day and walking to the local farmers market. Farmers from all over the Pikes Peak region come to Colorado Springs to sell their beautiful produce. I have never had more amazing cantaloupe, peaches and multicolored carrots than I had from the farmers market. The local foods movement is making a comeback the past few years. People want to connect with their food and want to know the farmers who grow their food. There are numerous reasons to eat locally, and by default, seasonally. Let's chat about it, shall we?!

Importance of Local Seasonal Eating

Environment & Sustainability

As you already know from chapter 3 on factory farms, you know that they are detrimental to the environment by contaminating the air and water supply. Did you know that big-ag farms that only grow produce are bad for the environment as well? The majority of the produce in supermarkets comes from huge farms which spray chemicals on the food which in turn get into our water system and air. Industrial farms, on the other hand, are detrimental to the environment by polluting the air, surface water, and groundwater, over-consuming fossil fuel and water resources, degrading soil quality, inducing erosion, and accelerating the loss of biodiversity. Not only does it harm the environment but industrial farms also harm the health of the workers and surrounding community by consistent exposure to pesticides. Many conventional foods travel on average 1,000-3,000 miles.

Unlike the industrial farms, local farms are primarily small and family run. Local farms typically utilize sustainable practices by using minimal to no pesticides, composting and non-till agriculture, minimized transportation to the markets and minimal to no packaging. Local farming also helps build a strong community. Farmers truly are the backbone of America, and really any country. When you get to know your farmers you are able to directly help them continue to prosper and feed the community.

I want to clarify that local and sustainable are not necessarily the same thing. You can live in a place where there is a large factory farm in your city. That farm would be local but by no means sustainable as we have discussed. So when searching for local farms to support in your area check out these resources: Localharvest.org

Good for the Body

Next time you are at the grocery store picking up produce take a look at where the produce is grown. Many times, especially during the winter, you will find berries from Chile, or grapes and tomatoes from Mexico. Once the produce is picked it starts to lose nutrients. Now imagine produce being shipped from out of the country, how many nutrients are lost! Crazy right? Produce found in large supermarkets spends either days or even weeks in a cold shipping container. On top of that, food that comes from far away is more susceptible to contamination.

When you shop local and support local farmers your body benefits because many times produce is picked right before they head over to the market. You get the freshest fruits and vegetables possible from right down the road. You will immediately taste the difference between a locally grown organic apple to an apple from across the country. Part of the reason produce that is grown locally tastes better is because the fruit or veggie has more time to ripen, yielding to a better-tasting food.

As a small business owner I love to see other local small businesses succeed and thrive. When you choose to spend your hard-earned money with a local farmer for produce instead of, say Wal-Mart, that money stays in the local economy. Let's look at it like this, if each dollar spent locally produces 2 times as much money for the local economy then we can double our buying power by purchasing only locally grown foods. So eating local can help harness our individual economic power and fight the global food industry.

It is so true, where and how consumers spend their money has a direct effect on our food supply. If we were all to spend our money on organic produce, purchase cruelty-free products only and not purchase meat, the corporations would listen, organic farmers would have more incentive to continue their sustainable practices, companies would stop testing on animals and there would be a tremendous decrease in farmed animals. Let's take control of our food system!

Where to Support Local Farms

It is farmer's market Saturday! I grab my re-useable bags and before I know it I am surrounded by the beauty of fresh local produce, new vegetables to try, the smell of fresh baked bread being sold and luxurious locally made olive oils to try. I love chatting it up with the farmers and getting to know them and what their farming practices are. If you live in an area of the country where there are not many farmers markets there are other ways to eat local through a community supported agriculture program or food cooperative.

Farmers Markets

Farmers markets are communal spaces in which multiple farmers gather to sell their farm products directly to consumers. When checking out the vendors at the market, chat them up. Get to know the farmers, how their produce is handled, and whether or not they use pesticides and chemicals on their plants. My advice for a successful farmers market trip is:

Walk the entire market and check out the prices of the produce. You may notice that organic lettuce may be more expensive than the commercial produce. However, you know that the organic farmer uses sustainable practices and a healthier crop for your body as well.

Get to the market as early as possible for the best selection of produce. Weekend markets are typically busier so if you want to beat the crowds and heat, and get the best selection, go first thing.

If you are looking for more deals go at the end of the market when farmers are willing to drop the price of produce to get rid of it.

Take cash! Although many vendors are now accepting credit cards with Square and similar systems, many still are not.

Get to know the farmers, have fun with the experience. Taste the produce before purchasing to make sure you like it.

Find a farmers market in your area:

http://www.ams.usda.gov/AMSv1.0/farmersmarkets

Community Supported Agriculture

CSAs are direct-to-consumer programs in which consumers

buy a "share" of a local farm's projected harvest. Consumers are often required to pay for their share of the harvest up front. In return you receive a weekly basket of goodies from the farmer's harvest. CSA participants often pick up their CSA shares in a communal location, or the shares may be delivered directly to customers. CSAs play an integral role in farm-to-community relationships. The CSA season generally lasts from late spring until early fall.

Find growers in your area who participate in community supported agriculture here:

http://www.nal.usda.gov/afsic/pubs/csa/csa.shtml

Community Gardens

Community gardens are becoming more and more popular in America. At a community garden you can plant your own produce along with others from the area. You are able to go to the garden and pick straight from the garden. The mission of a community garden is to bring members of the community together through food. Many of the community gardens you can find in urban and suburban settings where it may be more difficult to grow your own. Communities that have gardens see lower crime rates and increased property values. Community gardens also help heal the soil and environment, promote healthy bugs and wildlife, and more!

To find a community garden in your area be sure to visit

https://communitygarden.org/

Food Cooperatives

Food co-ops are formed by local community members who have a shared goal to provide low-cost healthy food to members of the co-op. Co-ops are similar to businesses except that they are owned by the members and are non-profit organizations. Each member gets a vote of how the co-op is run, making it a very democratic organization. Most food that co-ops sell local and organic so you know you are getting quality produce for your family.

To find a food cooperative in your area visit these sources:

http://www.coopdirectory.org/directory.htm

http://www.localharvest.org/food-coops/

Farms

Many local farms have programs where you can go to the farm on certain days and go out to the fields and pick your very own produce! Doesn't get any fresher than that! You can either pay for the produce you pick or you can work at the farm and buy your food that way. Either way it is a great way to connect with your food, community and soul.

Seasonal Produce

Winter

Acorn squash	Parsnips
Butternut squash	Sweet potatoes
Turnips	Purple & green cabbage
Collard greens	Broccoli
Swiss and rainbow chard	Kale
Brussels sprouts	Spinach
Carrots	Fennel
Cauliflower	Grapefruit
Celery root	Oranges
Pears	Leeks
Lemons	Persimmons

Spring

Asparagus	Mango
Strawberries	Limes
Arugula	Grapefruit
Fennel	Apricots
Artichokes	Radishes
Sugar snap peas	Jicama
Green beans	Honeydew

Summer

Beets	Cantaloupe
Butter (Bibb) lettuce	Cherries
Eggplant	Figs
Cucumbers	Grapes
Bell peppers	Nectarines
Okra	Peaches
Sugar snap peas	Pineapples
Summer squash	Plums
Swiss chard	Raspberries
Tomatoes	Watermelon
Zucchini	Strawberries
Blackberries	Blueberries

Fall

Acorn squash	Sweet potatoes
Arugula	Swiss chard
Endive	Cranberries
Brussels sprouts	Grapes
Butternut squash	Kumquats
Patty pan squash	Pears
Kale	Pomegranates
Pumpkin	Radicchio

Year Round

Bell peppers
Bok choy
Cabbage
Carrots
Celery
Celery root

Mushrooms
Onions
Avocados
Bananas
Lemons

What Happens Next?

Whatever your primary reason for beginning a vegan life, whether it be for the environment, health and/or the welfare of farmed animals, know that you rock! You are paving the way to a more compassionate and sustainable world. You can either transition to a vegan life cold turkey or gradually. There is no one right way to become vegan because everyone is different and each body is different.

This book is meant to be a guide for you, to help you become a vegan in a healthful way. I want for you all to feel vibrant and with more energy than ever before. When you follow the advice, information and tips provided in this book, transitioning to a vegan diet will be easier than ever!

I know that this was a lot of information to take in and I want you to know that I am not just going to throw this book at ya and be done with it. There are a variety of ways I am here to support you on your vegan journey.

I want to invite you to share your vegan journey, stories and questions with me. Join my Essential Vegan Facebook page at https://www.facebook.com/TheEssentialVegan or shoot me an email at Christina@forksnspoonsco.com, and subscribe to my monthly newsletter where you will be kept up to date on what is going on with Forks N' Spoons and receive recipes and tips for successful vegan living.

I want to leave you with a Sanskrit saying that I live my life by each day.

LOKAH SAMASTA SUKHINO BHAVANTU

May all creatures everywhere be happy and free and may the thoughts, words and actions of my own life contribute in some way to that happiness and to that freedom for all.

Chapter References

Chapter 3

Cancer

http://www.huffingtonpost.com/kathy-freston/vegan-diet-cancer_b_2250052.html

Heart health

http://www.peta.org/living/food/clean-clogged-arteries-vegan-diet/

http://www.webmd.com/diabetes/news/20081001/vegan-diet-good-type-2-diabetes

Depleting rainforest

http://www.peta.org/about-peta/faq/how-does-eating-meat-harm-the-environment/#ixzz2r9RWBQVw

http://www.peta.org/about-peta/faq/how-does-eating-meat-harm-the-environment/#ixzz2r9Rp6MDa

http://www.peta.org/about-peta/faq/how-does-eating-meat-harm-the-environment/#ixzz2r9RceJmU

Agriculture run-off

http://www.peta.org/about-peta/faq/how-does-eating-meat-harm-the-environment/#ixzz2r9RiSfub

http://www.vegetariantimes.com/article/the-environmental-impact-of-a-meat-based-diet/

http://www.nrdc.org/water/pollution/nspills.asp

http://www.peta.org/about-peta/faq/how-does-eating-meat-harm-the-environment/#ixzz2r9RxhteS

Chapter 4

Healthy heart

http://www.webmd.com/heart-disease/features/can-you-reverse-heart-disease

Arthritis

http://www.drfuhrman.com/disease/arthritis.aspx

Type 2 diabetes

http://www.pcrm.org/health/diabetes-resources/the-vegan-diet-how-to-guide-for-diabetes-step-1

About the Author

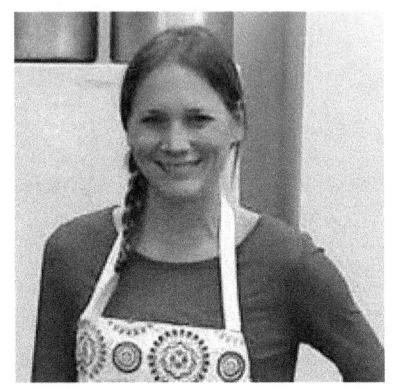

Christina Summers is the creator of Forks N' Spoons, an all vegan cooking school based out of Colorado Springs, Colorado teaching people to make vegan food easy and delicious.

Since 2012, Christina has guided people to live healthful lives with her Holistic Health Coaching Certification through the Institute of Integrative Nutrition. Christina's passion for healthy vegan living and food is contagious and she's eager to show others that living a vegan life is easier than ever.

When Christina is not teaching people how to live amazing vegan lives, she spends as much time as possible outdoors hiking, traveling and practicing yoga.

www.ingramcontent.com/pod-product-compliance
Lightning Source LLC
Chambersburg PA
CBHW070656290526
45790CB00001B/349